ALLE ZEIT WACH
1842

Psychological Treatment of Mental Illness

Research Strategies and Design

Edited by R. J. Daly and E. A. Sand

In Collaboration with Other Members
of the EMRC Study Group on Mental Illness Research
E. E. Anttinen, T. Helgason, H. Hippius and R. Sadoun

With 28 Figures and 22 Tables

Springer-Verlag
Berlin Heidelberg New York
London Paris Tokyo

Professor ROBERT J. DALY
Department of Psychiatry
Cork Regional Hospital
Wilton, Cork, Ireland

Professor E. ALFRED SAND
Laboratoire d'Epidémiologie
et de Médecine Sociale,
Ecole de Santé Publique,
Université Libre de Bruxelles
Campus Erasme 590/5,
B-1070 Bruxelles

ISBN-13: 978-3-642-72542-5 e-ISBN-13: 978-3-642-72540-1
DOI: 10.1007/978-3-642-72540-1

Library of Congress Cataloging-in-Publication Data. Psychological treatment of mental illness research and design. Contains the papers given at a symposium sponsored by the group of European Medical Research Councils in Brussels in May 1984. Includes bibliographies and index. 1. Psychotherapy – Research – Evaluation – Congresses. 2. Psychotherapy – Evaluation – Congresses. I. Daly, R.J. (Robert Joseph), 1936– . II. Sand, E.A. III. European Medical Research Councils. Study Group on Mental Illness Research. [DNLM: 1. Mental Disorders – therapy – congresses. 2. Psychotherapy – methods – congresses. WM 400 P9738 1984] RC337.P765 1987 616.89′1′072 87-12771

Softcover reprint of the hardcover 1st edition 1987

2125/3130-543210

European Science Foundation

This volume arises from the work of the Study Group on Mental Illness, a priority activity of the European Medical Research Councils (EMRC), which in turn is one of the five Standing Committees of the European Science Foundation (ESF). The EMRC, like the other ESF Committees, which cover the natural sciences, space science, humanities and the social sciences, brings together the research councils and academies of 18 European countries. Under the auspices of EMRC and ESF generally European scientists work on topics of common concern, co-ordinate the use of expensive facilities, and discover and define new endeavours that would benefit from a co-operative approach. Other typical work in the field studied in this book includes the European Training Programme in Brain and Behaviour Research, run by the ESF, closely linked with EMRC. In 1987 it brought together 500 youngs scientists from all over Europe in its Fellowships and residential courses.

Further information on EMRC and ESF activities can be obtained from:

European Science Foundation
1 Quai Lezay Marnésia
6700 Strasbourg, France

Foreword

The group of European Medical Research Councils (EMRC) was formed in 1971 by the medical research councils or equivalent organizations in Western Europe and became a Standing Committee of the European Science Foundation in 1975. The aims of the EMRC are to exchange information on research policies and to initiate and stimulate international cooperation in biomedical research.

Research on mental illness is one of the areas of special importance identified by the EMRC. Having surveyed the activities of its member organizations in mental illness research the EMRC decided in 1978 to set up a study group in order to promote European collaboration on research needed in this field. It was decided that emphasis should be on research on treatment and on the evaluation of treatment. The group prepared a proposal to the EMRC which suggested organizing small workshops with the participation of two or three research workers from each member country as well as from organizations with observer status in the EMRC such as they WHO and the National Institutes of Health in the United States. The members of the Study Group nominated by the EMRC are at present Professors E. Anttinen (Finland), R. Daly (Ireland), T. Helgason (Iceland; chairman), H. Hippius (Federal Republic of Germany), and E. A. Sand (Belgium), and Dr. R. Sadoun (France).

The purpose of the EMRC is to identify lacunae in present knowledge and to stimulate the international research activities needed to fill these lacunae. It is the hope of the study group that the questions that this volume raises will stimulate further research in the important field of psychological treatments of mental and physical illness.

The study group wants to acknowledge the support and interest of the member councils of the EMRC as well as the assistance of the European Science Foundation and its staff. Professors R. Daly and E. A. Sand undertook the arduous task of editing the volume. However, the book would not be available had it not been for the genuine interest and professional service given by the staff of Springer-Verlag.

Reykjavík, March 1987

Tómas Helgason
Chairman of the EMRC Study Group
on Mental Illness Research

Preface

This volume contains the papers given at a symposium sponsored by the group of European Medical Research Councils (EMRC) in Brussels in May 1984.

The EMRC meets annually to discuss the science policies and research activities being pursued by member organizations and to consider ways in which cooperation and collaboration can best be promoted. To achieve these aims it has set up a number of committees, one of which is the Study Group on Mental Illness Research. The Study Group has concerned itself with seeking to find priority areas for mental illness research and to interest member organizations in promoting research in areas where there are important lacunae.

Thus far the Study Group has held a series of international workshops on mental illness research with contributions from both Europe and the United States. This was the third in the series, which began with a workshop entitled *Methodology in Evaluation of Psychiatric Treatment* (Cambridge University Press, 1983), held in Vienna in June 1981. The second workshop was *The Long-term Treatment of Functional Psychoses* (Cambridge University Press, 1983) and was held in Viterbo in May 1983.

Methodological difficulties concerning psychotherapeutic treatments had emerged as a theme running through the first two workshops, hence the workshop on research strategies and design in psychological treatments of mental illness. The range of topics was confined to treatments involving adults, sick or disabled people. No attempt was made to cover milder neurotic disorders or problems such as obesity and smoking. Emphasis was placed on the methodology of evaluating psychological treatments.

The resulting papers amply demonstrate that methodologies *are* available which can reliably and validly evaluate psychological treatments. This is in sharp contrast to the widespread perception of this being a grey area where few conclusions can be drawn.

Both the consumer and the medical practitioner wish to see less reliance on drug treatments and greater availability of psychotherapies, but further investment in new treatments must be based on scientific evaluation.

R. J. Daly
E. A. Sand

Contents

List of Contributors

You will find the address of each first mentioned author at the beginning of the respective contribution

Evaluation Research on Psychotherapy in the Federal Republic of Germany *

D. von Zerssen [1], H.-J. Möller, and U. Baumann

Introduction

This is a brief survey of evaluation research on psychotherapy performed on psychiatric patients in the Federal Republic of Germany (FRG) after World War II, stressing work that has been published in German books or journals. The review excludes research undertaken in other German-speaking countries (German Democratic Republic, Austria, and Switzerland) because of the scantiness of relevant information available to the authors. The report is further restricted to psychological therapies in a technical sense, thus excluding many professional and non-professional activities such as counselling and rehabilitative measures. Moreover, the application of therapeutic techniques to individual social problems such as marital problems (Schindler et al. 1980), so-called analogue studies of non-patients (e.g. students with spider phobias) (cf. reviews by Baumann and Stieglitz 1983; Butollo 1980; Peterman 1979; Petermann and Dommel 1982) and, furthermore, psychological treatments of medical patients (Koch 1982), including those with so-called psychosomatic disorders (Beckmann et al. 1976; Rohrmeier 1982), are not considered here. The review is also not concerned with so-called process studies (see Kächele and Schors 1981) unless they were conducted in the context of outcome studies. Finally, the following topics are not dealt with: discussions of psychoanalytical theory from the point of view of the philosophical theory of science (Möller 1978; Thomä and Kächele 1973; Westmeyer 1976, 1978), and reviews of the general standards of research on psychotherapy (Baumann 1981; Enke et al. 1983; Hartig 1975; Köhnken et al. 1979; Minsel and Scheller 1983; Möller and Benkert 1980; Petermann 1977; Petermann and Hehl 1979; Reinecker 1983; Wittmann 1983), of methods of assessment and documentation (Baumann 1982; Baumann and Krüger 1982; Bommert and Hockel 1981; Möller and von Zerssen 1980; Rudolf 1980; Scholz 1982; Seidenstücker and Baumann 1978; von Zerssen 1979; Zielke 1982) and of statistical data analyses (Huber 1973; Krauth 1981; Petermann 1977; Rost 1982). Thus, the central aim will be to

* An updated German version of this article has been published by D. v. Zerssen, H.-J. Möller, U. Baumann, and G. Bühringer (1986) Evaluative Psychotherapieforschung in der Bundesrepublik Deutschland und West-Berlin. Psychother. Psychosom. Med. Psychol. 36:8-17

[1] Max-Planck-Institut für Psychiatrie, Kraepelinstraße 2, D-8000 München 40

Psychological Treatment of Mental Illness
Edited by R. J. Daly and E. A. Sand

summarize empirical evaluation of psychotherapeutic measures in psychiatric inpatients or outpatients. To make this survey of the literature more comprehensible for foreign readers an outline of the historical development and the professional organization of psychotherapy in the FRG is presented first.

Historical Background

Psychotherapy has a long-standing tradition in German-speaking countries. In Germany its development was partially interrupted during the Nazi era, particularly with respect to "orthodox" psychoanalytical treatment which had already been critically evaluated by Fenichel (1930) at the Berlin Psychoanalytic Institute. Many leading psychoanalysts such as Abraham, Alexander, Fenichel, and Hartmann emigrated from Germany after 1933, or even before that time. After World War II, a slow but steady recovery of psychotherapeutical training and activity could be observed, but almost two decades went by before serious research on the evaluation of psychotherapy was published in the German literature (de Boor and Künzler 1963; Cremerius 1962; Dührssen and Jorswieck 1965).

These investigations, in particular the Berlin study (Dührssen and Jorswieck 1965), stimulated the interest of health professionals in psychoanalytical work and prepared insurance companies for the acceptance of this type of therapy in ambulatory treatment by psychotherapists as financially compensable in 1967. Previously, only short-term psychotherapy on a pragmatic basis (relaxation, hypnosis and supportive psychotherapy) had been part of the medical health service. Psychoanalytic treatment, however, was provided only by a limited number of specially trained physicians and some psychologists in inpatient facilities or private practice.

During the late sixties a growing influence of psychological treatments, developed and applied, above all, by psychologists, could be observed in the care of psychiatric patients within the FRG. There were two main centres where this development began and where originally most evaluative studies were also executed: first, in Hamburg regarding Roger's non-directive (client-centred) psychotherapy (*Gesprächspsychotherapie;* Tausch 1981) and, secondly, in Munich with respect to behaviour therapy (Bergold and Selg 1970; Brengelmann and Tunner 1973). Since then, these therapies have been established at most institutes of clinical psychology at German universities. Psychoanalytical treatment and research, however, are preferred by physicians working in university psychiatric hospitals and particularly those employed in units of psychotherapy and/or psychosomatics (at all university hospitals in the FRG). The same applies to training in psychotherapy at these and other medical institutions (mental hospitals, psychiatric departments at community hospitals) and to the training of psychotherapeutically oriented physicians (mainly psychiatrists) in free practice. It is also true with respect to almost all psychotherapeutic training institutions where other psychiatrists and physicians are instructed, on a private basis, in the theory and practice of psychotherapy. These institutions belong to various psychoanalytic associations, mainly Freudian in orientation. Psychotherapeutic training of physicians is also given at conferences and courses, the latter particularly for relaxation techniques (autogenic Training; Schultz 1982). Instruction in the various therapeutic techniques of "humanistic psychology" (Gestalt therapy, transactional analysis, psychodrama, rational-emotive therapy, and others) by private organizations is also accessible to physicians, but is used much more by psychologists. These techniques seem to play a role only in the therapeutic activities of psychologists but so far have not elicited significant research on evaluating therapeutic success (see Baumann and Stieglitz 1983; Butollo 1980; Petermann 1979; Petermann and Dommel 1982).

Until now, the postwar development of psychotherapy research within the FRG, which followed that within the English-speaking countries with a delay of 8–10 years, has involved replication of results rather than being creative, although sometimes at a methodologically rather high level. Only a few major contributions to the theory and/or practice of psychotherapy and methods of evaluating its effectiveness are worth mentioning: in the theoretical field, Schulz-Hencke's neopsychoanalysis (see Schwidder 1959) and the anthropological foundation of psychotherapy by von Gebsattel (1959), which is a philosophical interpretation of psychopathological phenomena rather than a psychodynamic or other kind of psychological theory; in the field of psychotherapeutic techniques, the autogenic training mentioned above (Schultz 1982) and its combination with hypnotic techniques (*gestufte Aktivhypnose;* Kretschmer 1949), and a psychoanalytically oriented technique designated *katathymes Bilderleben* ("guided affective imagery"; Leuner 1980; Leuner and Lang 1982) which was derived from Kretschmer's technique of *Bildstreifendenken* (Kretschmer 1949); finally, in the field of behavioural therapy, a well-structured group training of assertive behaviour, the Assertiveness Training Programme (ATP; Ullrich and Ullrich de Muynck 1978; Ullrich de Muynck and Ullrich 1976), represents a new development. This technique also involves diagnostic assessment and evaluation of therapeutic success and has, indeed, stimulated a relatively large series of evaluation studies (Ullrich de Muynck et al. 1980).

Organization of Psychotherapeutic Services and Research

Most of the approximately 61.5 million inhabitats of the FRG belong to a health insurance company, either as members or by being close relatives of members. Health insurance has been mandatory (since 1911) for salaried employees, except for those above a certain income limit. The total number of members (including voluntary members) of the various kinds of companies amounted to 35.4 million people plus 21.5 million dependants in 1980. The government figure for members of private insurance companies was then

4.7 million (including dependants). It can be inferred that more than 95% of the population are insured by either mandatory or private companies. An additional 2% (consisting, for example, of policemen) receive free health care. Although the rules governing financial support of psychological treatment vary considerably in the case of private insurance companies, mandatory insurance has guaranteed full financial compensation for psychodynamic therapy under fairly well-defined conditions (since 1976 up to 50–80 sessions of psychodynamic therapy, either individual or group therapy, up to 120–150 sessions of analytic group therapy, and up to 240–300 sessions of individual psychoanalysis). In 1982 1700 psychoanalytically trained medical psychotherapists and 1110 non-medical psychoanalysts (predominantly psychologists) were engaged in an ambulatory service of this kind. There is a much higher number of specialists and non-specialists who offer analytical and other kinds of psychotherapy in various institutions (mainly psychiatric or psychotherapeutic clinics, including outpatient departments) or on a private basis in free practice. Moreover, pragmatic therapies (above all relaxation techniques and supportive psychotherapy) are applied by many physicians in free practice, and behaviour therapy, non-directive psychotherapy and other techniques are practised by clinical psychologists in psychiatric institutions, psychological institutes, other institutions and free practice. An unknown number of psychologists in free practice have signed a contract with an insurance company governing behavioural treatment (up to 60 or even 80 sessions per case).

According to an extensive survey (Fichter and Wittchen 1980; Wittchen and Fichter 1980), the total number of psychologists engaged in psychotherapeutic activities within the FRG was approximately 6000 in 1977. There were more than 2000 additional non-medical professionals (counsellors and others) who practised some kind of psychotherapy (in a broader sense). The total number of medical psychotherapists cannot be estimated on a comparable basis, but there must have been considerably more than the 1200 psychoanalysts known to exist at that time (compared with at least 1700 in 1982!; personal communication from the Kassenärztliche Bundesvereinigung, Cologne, November 1982). It may well be that, in all, an equal number of physicians and non-medical professionals have been trained in, and are applying, some type of psychotherapy. However, there is a rather uneven distribution of psychotherapeutic services between urban and rural areas and, within cities, between areas with marked socioeconomic differences (Fichter et al. 1983; Wittchen et al. 1980).

In relation to the growing influence of psychotherapy on medical and non-medical services for mental patients, the research activities in this field are rather limited and restricted mainly to university hospitals, psychological institutes at universities, and a small number of special research institutes (such as the Max-Planck-Institut für Psychiatrie in Munich). The funding of projects on the evaluation of psychotherapy is meagre compared with that of the evaluation of somatic treatments. In the field of psychopharmacology, a considerable amount of money is raised by pharmaceutical companies. Psychotherapeutic research, however, is almost exclusively supported by the narrow budgets of the institutions where it is performed, or by funds from the Deutsche Forschungsgemeinschaft, the Bundesministerium für Forschung und Technologie (Ministry of Research and Technology), or some other financially less solvent organization.

Methodology of Research

The methodology of research on the evaluation of psychotherapy within the FRG has profited considerably from the work of psychologists. New strategies and technologies, developed mainly in English-speaking countries, have been digested and critically evaluated in the German literature (e.g. Baumann 1984; Hartig 1975; Köhnken et al. 1979; Petermann and Hehl 1979). An evaluation technique developed in the FRG but so far used only for evaluating the success of rehabilitative measures in a single-case study is the technique of constructive behavioural measurement (*konstruktive Verhaltensmessung;* Frey et al. 1979). Moreover, quite a number of new self-rating scales have been constructed and proved useful in the evaluation of psychiatric treatment including psychotherapy (e.g. Beckmann and Richter 1975; Fahrenberg et al. 1978; Ullrich de Muynck and Ullrich 1976; von Zerssen and Koeller 1976). The methodological standards for evaluation research in psychiatry have been critically reviewed in a monograph (Biefang 1980a). The contributions to it, which are most pertinent to the evaluation of psychotherapy, were written by psychiatrists (Möller und Benkert 1980; von Zerssen and Möller 1980), psychiatrists and psychologists (e.g. von Cranach and Wittchen 1980), and a sociologist (Biefang 1980b). This cooperation of specialists from different fields has also proved most fruitful in empirical research on the evaluation of psychotherapy (e.g. Meyer 1981; Ullrich de Muynck et al. 1980).

Although during the seventies a growing number of outcome studies concerning psychoanalytic treatment were published in the FRG, it can be argued that a comparison of short-term psychotherapy with long-term psychoanalytic treatment has not yet been adequately performed (Kächele and Schors 1981). An objection to many studies of modes of treatment preferred by clinical psychologists (behaviour therapy, non-directive psychotherapy, etc.) is that they are of low clinical relevance because they have been performed only on very mildly disturbed subjects. Moreover, there is a lack of theory-related research in this area (Baumann and Stieglitz 1983). Common to these and psychoanalytic investigations is the lack of cost-benefit analyses, with some notable exceptions (e.g. Bühringer 1981; Koester et al. 1982; partially also Dührssen and Jorswieck 1965).

General Characteristics of Evaluation Studies in the German Literature

Apart from the great number of case reports (especially in the psychoanalytic literature) and follow-up investigations (see Göllner 1975), most psychotherapy studies have hitherto been conceptualized as global outcome studies. There is, however, a marked trend toward more informative designs describing the course of change during therapy and, in some studies, analysing process variables. Within this context, single-case studies using adequate statistical procedures have gained importance (Petermann and Hehl 1979). The main focus of psychotherapy research is now shifting from the simple question of the global effectiveness of psychotherapy to the following more complex one (Hartig 1975): What kind of therapy applied by what therapist under what conditions has what effects on what patient with what kind of problem and what are the reasons for this? This development is similar to tendencies in Anglo-American research which serves as a model for most of the psychotherapeutic studies in German-speaking countries. Recently, combined process-outcome studies have become the "ideal" research design in psychotherapy, an ideal which is fulfilled only in very few studies (similar to the situation in the English-speaking countries).

A survey of all empirical studies of psychotherapy (including those performed outside psychiatric and other medical institutions) that appeared in the German literature between 1976 and 1978 showed that there were 32 behaviour therapy studies, 13 psychoanalytic therapy studies, three studies of client-centred therapy, three of autogenic training and one of theme-centred interaction methods (Petermann 1979), among others. (It should be mentioned that this survey contained duplicate listings.) A similar distribution was announced in a survey of the German literature of the years from 1978 to 1981 (Petermann and Dommel 1982). Recently, more studies concerning autogenic training and especially client-centred therapy have been reported (Baumann and Stieglitz 1983).

Not taking into account special psychotherapeutic methods, the reports on empirical studies of psychotherapy can be structured according to different target symptoms and syndromes. It becomes apparent that studies of neurotic disorders are the most frequent, followed by those of psychosomatic diseases and addiction (Butollo 1980; Kächele 1981; Möller 1983; Petermann 1979; Thomä and Kächele 1983). This distribution can be partly explained by the general belief that neurotic and similar disorders should be the domain of psychotherapy. Consequently, it is not surprising that studies of endogenous psychoses and especially exogenic psychoses and psychogeriatric disturbances are rare. However, there is also a scarcity of reports on the psychotherapy of behavioural disturbances in childhood, which could be explained only by the low number of special institutions for child psychiatry in the FRG.

General problems of psychotherapy research in the FRG arise from the fact that most of the empirical studies are performed with rather small groups of patients, usually without adequate controls, and that mostly short-term therapies are evaluated. Studies that are more extensive or rigorous with regard to the number of patients, the duration of therapy, the inclusion of control groups, the incorporation of follow-up research, etc., are carried out very rarely. Although the methodological requirements of adequate psychotherapy research are known, financial restrictions hinder their realization.

Examples of Individual Studies

Structuring the following section around some of the most important studies conducted on various types of psychotherapy, we begin with psychoanalytic therapy. The early follow-up investigation by Dührssen and Jorswieck (1965) is of particular importance in spite of some methodological shortcomings. These authors analysed the duration of hospital stay within 5-year periods before and after a special type of psychoanalytical treatment (so-called dynamic psychotherapy) in about 120 outpatients with neurotic disorders and compared these data with those from a control group consisting of members of a general insurance company. The patients treated with psychotherapy showed a significant decrease in the duration of hospital stays, but there was no decrease in the duration of hospitalization in the other group.

As shown by the surveys of Kächele and Schors (1981) and Thomä and Kächele (1983), more recent studies of psychoanalytical outcome research are usually also follow-up studies or one-group studies without a control group, seldom use a standardized rating system and most often do not perform multipoint measurements (Deneke 1982; Engel et al. 1979; Ermann 1974; Göllner et al. 1978; Matussek and Triebel 1974; Petri and Thieme 1978; Pohlen and Bautz 1974; Rudolf 1980; Rüger 1976, 1981; Schwarz 1979; Wolfsteller and Kächele 1980). Control group designs with random assignment of patients are extremely rare in psychoanalytical research. The most important study in this respect is the Hamburg short-term psychotherapy comparison experiment (Meyer 1981) in which psychoanalytic focal therapy was compared with client-centred therapy in patients with functional disorders attending a psychosomatic outpatient unit. Enormous methodological efforts were made to describe and compare outcome and process variables and to analyse prognostic indicators. The main features of the study were: a rather large group of clinical patients ($n=88$), a large group of therapists, random assignment of patients to short-term psychotherapy or client-centred therapy (the mean duration of short-term psychotherapy being 26 ± 19 weeks and of client-centred therapy 18 ± 19 weeks), the inclusion of a waiting-list control group, standardized testing procedures, multiple outcome measures, four groups of independent assessors, three follow-up assessments within 3 years of therapy, use of process scales after each therapy session, and audio recording of all interviews, therapy sessions and follow-ups. The statistical analyses have not yet been completed, but the principal conclusion reached was that, measured by psychometric tests, the therapy groups showed a significantly more favourable outcome than the control group, the therapeutic effect being somewhat more pronounced in the client-centred therapy group than in the focal therapy group.

Studies of client-centred therapy have provided new techniques for the assessment of clients' therapeutic experiences by self-report. It was shown that there was a good correlation between self-report data and ratings by experts, based on the scales of Truax, and that self-report data concerning experiences during the first therapy session are of predictive value with respect to the outcome of psychotherapy. However, this is true not only of client-centred therapy but also of other types of psychotherapy (Eckert 1976; Eckert et al. 1977).

In a pilot study on the short-term effects of *katathymes Bilderleben* (guided affective imagery), Wächter and Pudel (1980a, b) compared the results obtained during 15 therapeutic sessions within 8 weeks in 14 psychiatric outpatients with data from an untreated control group. Using clinical judgement of improvement and changes in scale values of several questionnaires as measures of success, they found significantly more favourable results in the treatment group (see also Jung and Kulessa 1980; Kulessa and Jung 1979; Tress 1983).

From the very beginning behaviour therapy research has exhibited a strong empirical tendency. In addition to the usual group designs, different types of single-case experiment from simple ABA designs to complicated multiple-baseline designs have been performed. The studies have been intended to evaluate the effects of different elements of behaviour therapy, e.g. desensitization and flooding, particularly concerning the so-called monosymptomatic neuroses, or to examine the effects of complex therapy strategies such as training in self-assertiveness or social skills (Cohen et al. 1973; Fichter 1980; Hand and Tichatzky 1979; Heyse 1975; Kockott et al. 1975; Ullrich de Muynck and Ullrich 1976; Ullrich de Muynck et al. 1980, and others). It has been shown that behaviour therapy methods constitute effective treatment tools for neurotic disturbances, especially phobic disorders, compulsive disorders, anorexia nervosa, and other types of overt neurotic behaviour. It has also been concluded that simple therapy of the main symptom is not sufficient but that additional work on the social problems and deficiencies of the patient is imperative. Of these studies, those by Fichter on anorexia nervosa (Fichter 1980, 1981; Fichter and Keeser 1980) deserve mentioning in view of their elaborate experimental design and assessment methods. The evaluated treatment programme consisted of operant conditioning of eating behaviour and weight gain, desensitization of certain phobic reactions, and, in addition, self-assertiveness training in groups, thus showing modern behaviour therapy to be a rather complex approach to neurotic behaviour. The therapeutic outcome was analysed not only by means of group statistic but also on the basis of ABA designs, multiple-baseline designs, or other single-case evaluation methods. Inasmuch as one can judge from a non-controlled group design, the treatment programme as a whole proved to be effective for specifically anorexic symptoms, but not for general neurotic traits such as feelings of insufficiency, sexual anxieties and anancastic features. The therapeutic effects were not maintained in several patients after discharge from the hospital, as shown by a 3-year follow-up, indicating that the therapeutic programme needs not only to be extended to non-specific symptoms but also supplemented by aftercare (Fichter et al. 1982).

Studies of behaviour therapy for alcohol or drug addiction should also be mentioned (Cohen et al. 1980; de Jong and Bühringer 1978; de Jong and Henrich 1980; Koester et al. 1981, 1982; Olbrich et al. 1982; Vollmer and Kraemer 1982) in view of the great number of inpatients and outpatients examined and treated within these programmes. However, the methods of evaluation were not highly sophisticated in that they predominantly utilized only group statistics from multimodal assessments at different points of measurement and lacked control groups. It was generally concluded that the behaviour therapy programmes evaluated seemed to be effective for drug and alcohol addicts and that the therapeutic result was stable, as shown by follow-up assessments, in a certain percentage of patients.

The trend of combining group and single-case designs is well represented by studies of behavioural therapy in severely and, in many of the cases, chronically disturbed neurotic depressives by de Jong et al. (1981a, b, 1983; de Jong 1982). Three components of the programme, i.e. activity planning, social skill training and cognitive therapy, were evaluated in these studies. In the first study, 20 patients were randomly assigned to two experimental groups to whom the three components of the total therapy programme were applied according to different time schedules. The global outcome was compared with that of a matched control group of neurotic inpatients who had previously been treated with unspecific psychotherapy on the same ward. In the second study, 20 patients treated in two experimental groups – one of them in rather the same way as in the first study, the other by cognitive therapy alone – were compared with a waiting-list control group. Multimethod assessments, including more specific outcome criteria concerning the different components of the programme, differentiated group statistics and time-series analyses of single-case data, were performed at different times before, during and after therapy to gather as much information as possible about relatively specific as well as non-specific factors of the treatment programme. Among other outcome criteria, cognitions, activities and depressive psychopathology were rated by psychiatrists, nurses and the patients themselves. With regard to psychopathology, a videotape was produced during a standardized interview. The average duration of inpatient treatment was 14 weeks.

Marked general improvement of depression took place as a result of the treatment programme, the patients showing a significant improvement over the control groups. Although the time-series analyses showed that the cognitive treatment component was significantly effective in some cases, the results of single-case analyses and group statistical comparisons, especially in the second study, did not reveal the expected superiority of cognitive therapy but rather demonstrated that the other treatment components were more important. Nevertheless, even the group receiving purely cognitive therapy showed a better outcome than the control group. The correlation of data obtained during treatment with follow-up data indicated that the amelioration of cognitive measures at the end of the therapy programme was related to a relatively long-lasting therapeutic effect, whereas the amelioration of activity and social skill measures resulted in less stable effects (de Jong et al. 1981a, b; de Jong 1982). Personality measures taken on admission proved to be of predictive value, neurotic traits, including "oral" dependency and low extroversion, indicating poor success (de Jong 1982).

An extensive investigation of the comparative effectiveness of three modifications of the Masters and Johnson technique for the treatment of couples with disturbed sexual relations was conducted by Arentewicz and Schmidt (1980). The resulting success rate proved independent of the number of therapists and the frequency of sessions in the three settings under comparison – a result which seems relevant from an economic point of view for planning treatments of this kind.

Behaviour therapy approaches have been evaluated not only in neurotic and related disorders but also in psychoses. The number of important studies on this subject, however, is quite small. The study by Cohen et al. (1973) is well known. They examined the effect of a token economy programme on chronic schizophrenic inpatients, using a simple ABA design without a control group and documenting only the amount of tokens and simple behavioural observation and psychopathological rating data. The analysis of the multi-measure assessment showed that, during the phase of contingent reinforcement of desired working behaviour, the expected amelioration of working behaviour actually took place. It was specific insofar as other social behaviours as well as the patients' psychopathology remained unchanged.

Of late, the interest of behaviour therapists has turned to social skills training or more complex therapy strategies in the treatment of schizophrenic patients. The most important study in this field appears to be that by Brenner et al. (1980a, b, 1982; see also Brenner et al. 1983) who combined social skills training with training in cognitive functions such as cognitive differentiation and social perception, thus following modern theories of basic disturbances of schizophrenic patients. The results of the methodologically excellent study of about 70 patients showed a great improvement in the experimental group compared with both an attention-control group and a simple control group. The differential analyses showed that the non-paranoid schizophrenics in particular benefited from cognitive training, a differentiation which was also seen at the follow-up 18 months later. On this basis, a differential indication was evaluated in a new study (Brenner et al. 1982).

A study comparing changes during behaviour therapy and client-centred therapy in phobic disorders (Grawe 1976; Plog 1976) is worth mentioning because of its differentiated statistical design. About 50 outpatients with phobic disturbances were randomly assigned to three groups: a behaviour therapy group, a client-centred therapy group, and an untreated control group. The patients were treated at one or two sessions a week for 6 months and followed up 4 months after the termination of psychotherapy. A standardized multimethod assessment was used, with several measurement times before, during and after the therapy programme. Group statistics served to evaluate global as well as differential outcome and outcome predictors. There was a significant improvement in the global outcome of the therapy groups as compared with the control group, but the differences in global outcome between the two psychotherapy groups were small. Above all, the expected advantage of behaviour therapy in reducing symptoms and of client-centred therapy in inducing more marked changes in personality traits did not appear in the data. Patients who were suffering most from phobic symptoms before therapy experienced the most intensive symptom reduction and, along with it, the best general improvement. Patients with low initial values of phobic symptoms did not experience significant therapeutic effects of behaviour therapy; in client-centred therapy, there was, however, no relationship between pretreatment scores of phobic symptomatology and therapy results. There were important differences in the pattern of change between the two treatments. In behaviour therapy, for example, there was a close relationship between symptom reduction and change in other aspects such as personality traits; in client-centred therapy there was only a weak correlation between change in symptomatology and in personality traits. Moreover, the degree of improvement showed a significantly more pronounced variation after behaviour therapy than after client-centred therapy – a finding which might be of general importance for evaluation research on psychotherapy where, so far, attention has focused on mean outcome values and has disregarded the scatter of individual values around it (Grawe 1981).

Final Comments

Comparative studies of basically different psychotherapeutic approaches are virtually lacking in the German literature. This applies to treatment of comparable cases on an inpatient or outpatient basis, and to basically different modes of treatment, e.g. psychotherapy in a technical sense compared with psychological management of the common sense type and/or active rehabilitative measures, with drug treatment, or with a combination of pharmacological and psychological therapy (a notable exception is Ullrich et al. 1975). In particular, comparative studies with long-term follow-up of at least 1–2 years have rarely been conducted and epidemiological intervention studies have not yet been undertaken. Family therapy is practised and propagated by some of the leading psychoanalysts in the FRG (see Richter 1974) and teaching in the various techniques and their theoretical foundation is provided at several training centres, but so far no evaluation studies have been carried out in this field. As already mentioned, cost-benefit analyses are usually neglected in German investigations.

Although the need for such investigations is fairly well recognized, there is not only a lack of financial support when it comes to realizing them but also a lack of motivation as well as competence on the part of therapists. It will be the task of the future both to make more funds available for this kind of research and to motivate and train psychotherapists to cooperate adequately with methodologists. The chances of a respectable performance of evaluation research on psychotherapy will largely depend on this collaboration of specialists in the therapeutic area, on the one hand, with specialists in the methodological field (mainly psychologists, but in certain projects also sociologists, economists, statisticians, and the like), on the other. This would serve as the best guarantee of scientific quality as well as of clinical relevance of this kind of research.

Appendix: Medical Institutions where Extensive Research on the Evaluation of Psychotherapy is Performed

1. Abteilung für Psychotherapie der Universität Ulm (Department of Psychotherapy at the University of Ulm): Among other projects, assessment of the success of psychoanalytic treatment, language content analysis of psychoanalytic treatment (Grünzig and Kächele 1978; Kächele and Mergenthaler 1981; Wolfsteller and Kächele 1980)
2. Forschungsstelle für Psychotherapie (Centre for Psychotherapy Research), Stuttgart: Among other studies, research on psychoanalytic group psychotherapy (Enke and Lermer 1978; Ermann 1974; Ermann and Ermann 1976; Göllner et al. 1978)
3. Forschungsstelle für Psychopathologie der Max-Planck-Gesellschaft (Institute for Psychopathology Research of the Max Planck Society), Munich: Research on psychoanalytic therapy of neuroses and especially psychoses (Matussek and Triebel 1974; Pohlen and Bautz 1974; Schwarz 1979)
4. Max-Planck-Institut für Psychiatrie (Max Planck Institute of Psychiatry), Munich: Research on behaviour therapy, e.g. in alcohol or drug addiction, anorexia nervosa, neurotic disorders, sexual disorders, and in brain-damaged or autistic children (de Jong and Bühringer 1978; Fichter 1980; Heyse 1975; Kockott et al. 1975; Ullrich de Muynck and Ullrich 1976; Vollmer and Kraemer 1982)
5. Psychiatrische Klinik, Psychosomatische Klinik, Psychologisches Institut der Universität Hamburg (Psychiatric Clinic, Psychosomatic Clinic and Psychological Institute of the University of Hamburg), to a certain extent working together in the Sonderforschungsbereich für psychosomatische Medizin der Universität Hamburg (Centre for Research on Psychosomatic Medicine at the University of Hamburg): Evaluation of psychoanalytic

short-term therapy and client-centred psychotherapy in psychosomatic patients, evaluation of behaviour therapy in compulsive disorders, differential evaluation of behaviour therapy in phobic disorders, analysis of process variables such as patients' experiences in psychotherapy and language analysis of psychotherapy (Dahme 1977; Eckert et al. 1977; Grawe 1976; Hand and Tichatzky 1979; Meyer 1981; Plog 1976; Schöfer 1977)
6. Psychotherapeutische Klinik der Universität Berlin (Psychotherapeutic Clinic of the University of Berlin): Catamnestic and other evaluations of psychoanalytic therapy (Dührssen and Jorswieck 1965; Dührssen 1972; Rudolf 1980)
7. Sonderforschungsbereich für vergleichende Forschung in der Nervenheilkunde und in der Psychosomatik der Universität Gießen (Centre for Comparative Research on Neurology and Psychosomatic Medicine at the University of Gießen): Research on patient–therapist interaction, automated analysis of verbal behaviour in psychotherapeutic situations (Beckmann et al. 1976; Brähler 1978; Brähler et al. 1974; Richter and Wirth 1978)
8. Zentralinstitut für Seelische Gesundheit (Centre for Mental Health), Mannheim: Research on behaviour therapy strategies in the treatment of chronic schizophrenia (Brenner et al. 1980a, b)

References

Arentewicz G, Schmidt G (eds) (1980) Sexuell gestörte Beziehungen. Springer, Berlin Heidelberg New York

Baumann U (1981) Differentielle Therapiestudien und Indikation. In: Baumann U (ed) Indikation zur Psychotherapie. Urban & Schwarzenberg, München, pp 199–209

Baumann U (1982) Dokumentation in der Psychotherapie. In: Baumann U, Berbalk H, Seidenstücker G (eds) Klinische Psychologie. Huber, Bern, pp 149–176 (Trends in Forschung und Praxis, vol 5)

Baumann U(ed) (1984) Psychotherapie: Makro-/Mikroperspektive. Hogrefe, Göttingen

Baumann U, Krüger, G (1982) Merkmalszusammenstellung für Psychotherapiedokumentation. In: Baumann U, Berbalk H, Seidenstücker G (eds) Klinische Psychologie. Huber, Bern, pp 177–185 (Trends in Forschung und Praxis, vol 5)

Baumann U, Stieglitz RD (1983) Psychotherapieforschung – Schwerpunkt psychologische Methoden. In: Häfner H (ed) Forschung für die seelische Gesundheit. Eine Bestandsaufnahme der psychiatrischen, psychotherapeutischen und psychosomatischen Forschung und ihre Probleme in der Bundesrepublik Deutschland. Springer, Berlin Heidelberg New York, pp 174–189

Beckmann D, Richter HE (1975) Gießen-Test. Huber, Bern

Beckmann D, Berger F, Leister G, Stephanos S (1976) A 4-year follow-up study of in-patient psychosomatic patients. Psychother Psychosom 27:168–178

Bergold J, Selg H (1970) Verhaltenstherapie. In: Schraml WJ (ed) Klinische Psychologie. Huber, Bern, pp 270–309

Biefang S (ed) (1980a) Evaluationsforschung in der Psychiatrie: Fragestellungen und Methoden. Enke, Stuttgart

Biefang S (1980b) Evaluationsforschung in Medizin und Gesundheitswesen. In: Biefang S (ed) Evaluationsforschung in der Psychiatrie: Fragestellungen und Methoden. Enke, Stuttgart, pp 7–53

Bommert H, Hockel M (eds) (1981) Therapieorientierte Diagnostik. Kohlhammer, Stuttgart

Boor C de, Künzler E (1963) Die psychosomatische Klinik und ihre Patienten (Erfahrungsbericht der Psychosomatischen Uni-Klinik Heidelberg). Klett, Stuttgart

Brähler E (1978) Die Erfassung des Interventionsstils von Therapeuten durch die automatische Sprachanalyse. Z Psychosom Med Psychoanal 24:156–168

Brähler E, Overbeck G, Braun D, Junker H (1974) Was kann die automatische Analyse des Sprech-Pausen-Verhaltens (on-off-pattern) von Arzt und Patient für die Beurteilung von Psychotherapien leisten? Z Psychosom Med Psychoanal 20:148–163

Brengelmann JC, Tunner W (eds) (1973) Behaviour therapy – Verhaltenstherapie. Urban & Schwarzenberg, München

Brenner HD, Seeger G, Stramke WG (1980a) Evaluation eines spezifischen Therapieprogramms zum Training kognitiver und kommunikativer Fähigkeiten in der Rehabilitation chronisch schizophrener Patienten in einem naturalistischen Feldexperiment. In: Hautzinger M, Schultz W (eds) Klinische Psychologie und Psychotherapie, vol 4. GWG DGVT, Cologne, pp 31–47

Brenner HD, Stramke WG, Mewes J, Liese F, Seeger G (1980b) Erfahrungen mit einem spezifischen Therapieprogramm zum Training kognitiver und kommunikativer Fähigkeiten in der Rehabilitation chronisch schizophrener Patienten. Nervenarzt 51:106–112

Brenner HD, Stramke W, Brauchli B (1982) Integriertes psychologisches Therapieprogramm bei chronisch schizophrenen Patienten: Untersuchungen zu Differentialindikation. In: Helmchen H, Linden M, Rüger U (eds) Psychotherapie in der Psychiatrie. Springer, Berlin Heidelberg New York, pp 77–85

Brenner HD, Rey E-R, Stramke WG (eds) (1983) Empirische Schizophrenieforschung. Huber, Bern

Bühringer G (1981) Planung, Steuerung und Bewertung von Therapieeinrichtungen für junge Drogen- und Alkoholabhängige. Röttger, München

Butollo W (1980) Behavior therapy in the German-speaking countries. Germ J Psychol 4:247–262

Cohen R, Florin I, Grusche A, Meyer-Osterkamp S, Sell H (1973) Dreijährige Erfahrungen mit einem Münzsystem auf einer Station für extrem inaktive, chronisch schizophrene Patienten. Z Klin Psychol 2:243–277

Cohen R, Appelt H, Eckert A, Olbricht R, Watzl H (1980) Erfahrungen mit einem verhaltenstherapeutischen Programm für alkoholkranke Frauen. In: Haase HJ (ed) Psychotherapie im Wirkungsbereich des psychiatrischen Krankenhauses. Perimed, Erlangen, pp 59–86

Cranach M von, Wittchen H-U (1980) Epidemiologische Aspekte der Evaluationsforschung in der psychiatrischen Versorgung. In: Biefang S (ed) Evaluationsforschung in der Psychiatrie: Fragestellungen und Methoden. Enke, Stuttgart, pp 208–249

Cremerius J (1962) Die Beurteilung des Behandlungserfolges in der Psychotherapie. Springer, Berlin Göttingen Heidelberg

Dahme B (1977) Zeitreihenanalyse und psychotherapeutischer Prozeß. In: Petermann F (ed) Methodische Grundlagen klinischer Psychologie. Beltz, Weinheim, pp 169–192

Deneke FW (1982) Analytische Gruppentherapie. Vandenhoeck & Ruprecht, Göttingen

Dührssen A (1972) Analytische Psychotherapie in Theorie, Praxis und Ergebnissen. Vandenhoeck & Ruprecht, Göttingen

Dührssen A, Jorswieck E (1965) Eine empirisch-statische Untersuchung zur Leistungsfähigkeit psychoanalytischer Behandlung. Nervenarzt 36:166–169

Eckert J (1976) Zur Prognose von psychotherapeutischen Effekten bei unterschiedlichen Behandlungsmethoden. Z Klin Psychol 5:153–163

Eckert J, Schwartz H-J, Tausch R (1977) Klienten-Erfahrungen und Zusammenhang mit psychischen Änderungen in personenzentrierter Gesprächspsychotherapie. Z Klin Psychol 6:177–184

Engel K, Rad M von, Becker H, Bräutigam W (1979) Das Heidelberger Katamneseprogramm. Med Psychol 5:124–137

Enke H, Lermer S (1978) Selbsterleben von Gruppenmitgliedern im Spiegel empirischer Untersuchungsbefunde. Prax Psychother 23:13–25

Enke H, Tschuschke V, Volk W (eds) (1983) Psychotherapeutisches Handeln. Kohlhammer, Stuttgart

Ermann M (1974) Verlaufsbeobachtung zur körperlichen Symptomatik bei stationär behandelten Neurotikern. Z Psychosom Med Psychoanal 20:378–383

Ermann M, Ermann G (1976) Differentialindikation im klinischen Feld. Z Psychosom Med Psychoanal 22:342–355

Fahrenberg J, Selg H, Hampel R (1978) Freiburger Persönlichkeitsinventar, FPI, 3rd ed. Hogrefe, Göttingen

Fenichel O (1930) Statistischer Bericht über die therapeutische Tätigkeit 1920–1930. In: 10 Jahre Berliner Psychoanalytisches Institut, Wien, pp 13–19

Fichter MM (1980) Klinische Verlaufsuntersuchungen zur Verhaltenstherapie der Pubertätsmagersucht. In: Hautzinger M, Schulz W (eds) Klinische Psychologie und Psychotherapie, vol 3. GWG DGVT, Berlin, pp 267–276

Fichter MM (1981) Zur Verhaltenstherapie und Prognose der Pubertätsmagersucht. In: Meermann R (ed) Anorexia nervosa. Enke, Stuttgart, pp 238–253

Fichter MM, Keeser W (1980) Behavioral treatment of an anorexic male: experimental analysis of generalization. Behav Anal Modif 4:152–168

Fichter MM, Wittchen H-U (1980) „Nicht-ärztliche" Psychotherapie im In- und Ausland. Zur psychotherapeutischen Versorgung durch nicht-ärztliche Berufsgruppen. Beltz, Weinheim

Fichter MM, Doerr P, Pirke KM, Lund R (1982) Behavior, attitude, nutrition and endocrinology in anorexia nervosa: longitudinal study in 24 patients. Acta Psychiatr Scand 66:429–444

Fichter MM, Weyerer S, Wittchen H-U, Dilling H (1983) Psychotherapy services and the prevalence of mental disorders in urban and rural areas. Arch Psychiatr Nervenkr 233:39–57

Frey S, Zerssen D von, Hansen W, Harders S (1979) Probleme der Verhaltensmessung in Einzelfalluntersuchungen. In: Petermann F, Hehl F-J (eds) Einzelfallanalyse. Urban & Schwarzenberg, München, pp 159–182

Gebsattel VE von (1959) Gedanken zu einer anthropologischen Psychotherapie. In: Frankl VE, Gebsattel VE von, Schultz JH (eds) Spezielle Psychotherapie I. Urban & Schwarzenberg, München, pp 531–567 (Handbuch der Neurosenlehre und Psychotherapie, vol 3)

Göllner R (1975) Was sagen katamnestische Untersuchungen über die Effektivität stationärer psychotherapeutischer Behandlungsmaßnahmen aus? In: Bericht über die Lage der Psychiatrie in der Bundesrepublik Deutschland – Zur psychiatrischen und psychotherapeutisch/psychosomatischen Versorgung der Bevölkerung. (Deutscher Bundestag, 7. Wahlperiode, Drucksache 7/4201) Bonner Universitäts-Buchdruckerei, Bonn, pp 921–941

Göllner R, Volk W, Ermann M (1978) Analyse von Behandlungsergebnissen eines zehnjährigen Katamneseprogramms. In: Beese F (ed) Stationäre Psychotherapie. Modifiziertes psychoanalytisches Behandlungsverfahren und therapeutisch nutzbares Großgruppengeschehen. Verlag für Medizinische Psychologie, Göttingen, pp 288–301

Grawe K (1976) Differentielle Psychotherapie. I. Huber, Bern

Grawe K (1981) Vergleichende Psychotherapieforschung. In: Minsel W-R, Scheller R (eds) Brennpunkte der Klinischen Psychologie, vol 1. Kösel, München, pp 149–183

Grünzig H-J, Kächele H (1978) Zur Differenzierung psychoanalytischer Angstkonzepte. Ein empirischer Beitrag zur automatischen Klassifikation klinischen Materials. Z Klin Psychol 7:1–17

Hand I, Tichatzky M (1979) Behavioral group therapy for obsessions and compulsions: first results of a pilot study. In: Sjödén P-O, Bates S, Dockens III WS (eds) Trends in behavior therapy. Academic, New York, pp 269–297

Hartig M (1975) Probleme und Methoden der Psychotherapieforschung. Urban & Schwarzenberg, München

Heyse H (1975) Response prevention and modelling in the treatment of obsessive-compulsive neurosis: a study of 24 patients. In: Brengelmann JC (ed) Progress in behavior therapy. Springer, Berlin Heidelberg New York, pp 53–58

Huber HP (1973) Psychometrische Einzelfalldiagnostik. Beltz, Weinheim

Jong R de (1982) Neurotische Depression und die Wirksamkeit psychologischer Therapie. Habilitationsschrift, Universität München

Jong R de, Bühringer G (eds) (1978) Ein verhaltenstherapeutisches Stufenprogramm zur stationären Behandlung von Drogenabhängigen. Röttger, München

Jong R de, Henrich G (1980) Follow-up results of a behavior modification program for juvenile drug addicts. Addict Behav 5:49–57

Jong R de, Ferstl R, Henrich G, Treiber R (1981a) Der Einfluß eines Verhaltenstherapieprogramms auf Therapieindikatoren bei neurotisch-depressiven Patienten. In: Michaelis W (ed) Bericht über den 32. Kongreß der Deutschen Gesellschaft für Psychologie in Zürich 1980, vol 2. Hogrefe, Göttingen, pp 581–584

Jong R de, Henrich G, Ferstl R (1981b) A behavioral treatment programme for neurotic depression. Behav Anal Modif 4:275–287

Jong R de, Henrich G, Treiber R (1983) Die Effekte von zwei psychologischen Therapien bei schwer neurotisch depressiven Patienten. In: Brengelmann JC, Bühringer G (eds): Therapieforschung für die Praxis, vol 3. Röttger, München, pp 117–139

Jung F, Kulessa C (1980) Katamnestische Untersuchung einer 20-Stunden-Therapie mit dem Katathymen Bilderleben – Eine testpsychologische Studie. In: Leuner H (ed) Katathymes Bilderleben. Ergebnisse in Theorie und Praxis. Huber, Bern, pp 172–185

Kächele H, Schors R (1981) Ansätze und Ergebnisse psychoanalytischer Therapieforschung. In: Baumann U, Berbalk H, Seidenstücker G (eds) Klinische Psychologie. Huber, Bern, pp 209–257 (Trends in Forschung und Praxis, vol 4)

Kächele H, Mergenthaler E (eds) (1981) Computer-aided analysis of psychotherapeutic discourse. Ulm Psychotherapy Text Archive, Ulm

Koch U (1982) Psychotherapie im medizinischen Bereich. In: Baumann U, Berbalk H, Seidenstücker G (eds) Klinische Psychologie. Huber, Bern, pp 188–227 (Trends in Forschung und Praxis, vol 5)

Kockott G, Dittmar F, Nusselt L (1975) Systematic desensitization of erectile impotence: a controlled study. Arch Sex Behav 4:493–500

Köhnken G, Seidenstücker G, Baumann U (1979) Zur Systematisierung von Methodenkriterien für Psychotherapiestudien. In: Baumann U, Berbalk H, Seidenstücker G (eds) Klinische Psychologie. Huber, Bern, pp 72–128 (Trends in Forschung und Praxis, vol 2)

Koester W, Schneider R, Hachmann E, Mai N (1981) Dokumentation und Evaluation der stationären Behandlung von Alkohol- und Medikamentenabhängigen nach einem verhaltenstherapeutischen Programm – Beschreibung des Dokumentationssysstems und Ergebnisse. Suchtgefahren 27:193–206

Koester W, Schneider R, Hachmann E, Mai N (1982) Ergebnisse des stationären verhaltenstherapeutischen Programms zur Behandlung von Alkohol- und Medikamentenabhängigen: Katamnesen nach einem Jahr. In: Schneider R (ed) Stationäre Behandlung von Alkoholabhängigen. Röttger, München, pp 215–243

Krauth, J (1981) Statistische Methoden zur Veränderungsmessung. In: Baumann U, Berbalk H, Seidenstücker G (eds) Klinische Psychologie. Huber, Bern, pp 98–131 (Trends in Forschung und Praxis, vol 4)

Kretschmer E (1949) Psychotherapeutische Studien. Thieme, Stuttgart

Kulessa C, Jung FG (1979) Die Effizienz einer 20stündigen Kurzpsychotherapie mit dem Katathymen Bilderleben. Eine testpsychologische Untersuchung. Z Psychosom. Med Psychoanal 25:274–293

Leuner H (ed) (1980) Katathymes Bilderleben. Ergebnisse in Theorie und Praxis. Huber, Bern

Leuner H, Lang O (eds) (1982) Psychotherapie mit dem Tagtraum. Katathymes Bilderleben. Ergebnisse II: Fallanalysen, Theorie. Huber, Bern
Matussek P, Triebel A (1974) Die Wirksamkeit der Psychotherapie bei 44 Schizophrenen. Nervenarzt 45:569–575
Meyer A-E (ed) (1981) The Hamburg short psychotherapy comparison experiment. Psychother Psychosom 35
Minsel WR, Scheller R (eds) (1983). Brennpunkte der Klinischen Psychologie. Forschungskonzepte der Klinischen Psychologie, vol 6. Kösel, München
Möller HJ (1978) Psychoanalyse – erklärende Wissenschaft oder Deutungskunst? Fink, München
Möller HJ (1983) Psychologische und soziale Aspekte in der klinisch-psychiatrischen Forschung. Forschungsaktivitäten in der BRD in ihrer Beziehung zur internationalen Forschung. In: Häfner H (ed) Forschung für die seelische Gesundheit. Springer, Berlin Heidelberg New York, pp 98–118
Möller H-J, Benkert O (1980) Methoden und Probleme der Beurteilung der Effektivität psycho-pharmakologischer und psychologischer Therapieverfahren. In: Biefang S (ed) Evaluationsforschung in der Psychiatrie: Fragestellungen und Methoden. Enke, Stuttgart, pp 54–128
Möller H-J, Zerssen D von (1980) Probleme und Verbesserungsmöglichkeiten der psychiatrischen Diagnostik. In: Biefang S (ed) Evaluationsforschung in der Psychiatrie: Fragestellungen und Methoden. Enke, Stuttgart, pp 167–207
Olbrich R, Cohen R, Watzl H (1982) Verhaltenstherapie bei alkoholkranken Frauen: Resümierende Bemerkungen am Ende eines 6jährigen stationären Modellversuches. In: Helmchen H, Linden M, Rüger U (eds) Psychotherapie in der Psychiatrie. Springer, Berlin Heidelberg New York, pp 220–224
Petermann F (ed) (1977) Psychotherapieforschung, Beltz, Weinheim
Petermann F (1979) Psychotherapie research. Germ J Psychol 3:168–186
Petermann F, Dommel N (1982) Psychotherapy research: current trends. Germ J Psychol 6:69–81
Petermann F, Hehl F-J (eds) (1979) Fortschritte der Klinischen Psychologie, Einzelfallanalyse, vol 18. Urban & Schwarzenberg, München
Petri H, Thieme E (1978) Katamnese zur analytischen Psychotherapie im Kindes- und Jugendalter. Psyche 32:21–51
Plog U (1976) Differentielle Psychotherapie II. Huber, Bern
Pohlen M, Bautz M (1974) Gruppenanalyse als Kurzpsychotherapie. Eine empirische Vergleichsuntersuchung bei spezifisch inhomogenen Gruppen von Psychotikern und Neurotikern. Nervenarzt 45:514–533
Reinecker H (1983) Grundlagen und Kriterien verhaltenstherapeutischer Forschung. AVM, Salzburg
Richter H-E (1974) Patient Familie. Rowohlt, Reinbek bei Hamburg
Richter H-E, Wirth H (1978) 7 Jahre Erfahrung mit der analytischen Zwei-Wochen-Paartherapie. Familiendynamik 3:20–46
Rohrmeier F (1982) Langzeiterfolge psychosomatischer Therapien. Springer, Berlin Heidelberg New York
Rost J (1982) Testtheoretische Modelle für die klinisch-psychologische Forschung und Diagnostik. In: Baumann U, Berbalk H, Seidenstücker G (eds) Klinische Psychologie. Huber, Bern, pp 58–110 (Trends in Forschung und Praxis, vol 5)
Rudolf G (1980) Wie messen sich Krankheit und Gesundheit in einem standardisierten Befund? Ergebnisse einer katamnestischen Untersuchung nach dynamischer Psychotherapie. Prax Psychother Psychosom 25:153–162
Rüger U (1976) Ergebnisse einer katamnestischen Nachuntersuchung an 21 Patienten fünf Jahre nach Abschluß einer ambulanten Gruppentherapie. Gruppenther Gruppendyn 10:313–330
Rüger U (1981) Stationär-ambulante Gruppenpsychotherapie. Springer, Berlin Heidelberg New York

Schindler L, Hahlweg K, Revenstorf D (1980) Partnerschaftsprobleme: Möglichkeiten zur Bewältigung. Springer, Berlin Heidelberg New York

Schöfer G (1977) Erfassung affektiver Veränderungen im Psychotherapieverlauf durch die Gottschalk-Gleser-Inhaltsanalyse. Z Klin Psychol Psychother 25:203–218

Scholz OB (1982) Interaktionsdiagnostik. In: Baumann U, Berbalk H, Seidenstücker G (eds) Klinische Psychologie. Huber, Bern, pp 112–148 (Trends in Forschung und Praxis, vol 5)

Schultz IH (1982). Das autogene Training (konzentrative Selbstentspannung), 17th ed. Thieme, Stuttgart

Schwarz F (1979) Ergebnisse nach stationärer Gruppenpsychotherapie neurotisch depressiver und zwangsneurotischer Patienten. Nervenarzt 50:379–386

Schwidder W (1959) Neopsychoanalyse (Harald Schultz-Hencke). In: Frankl VE, Gebsattel VE von, Schultz JH (eds) Spezielle Psychotherapie I. Urban & Schwarzenberg, München, pp 171–220 (Handbuch der Neurosenlehre und Psychotherapie, vol 3)

Seidenstücker G, Baumann U (1978) Multimethodale Diagnostik. In: Baumann U, Berbalk H, Seidenstücker G (eds) Klinische Psychologie. Huber, Bern, pp 134–182 (Trends in Forschung und Praxis, vol 1)

Tausch R (1981) Gesprächspsychotherapie, 8th ed. Hogrefe, Göttingen

Thomä H, Kächele H (1973) Wissenschaftstheoretische und methodologische Probleme der klinisch-psychoanalytischen Forschung. Psyche 27:159–173, 205–236, 309–355

Thomä H, Kächele H (1983) Bemerkungen zur Lage der psychoanalytischen Forschung in der BRD. In: Häfner H (ed) Forschung für die seelische Gesundheit. Springer, Berlin Heidelberg New York, pp 159–173

Tress W (1983) Psychotherapeutische Verläufe. Enke, Stuttgart

Ullrich R, Ullrich de Muynck R (eds) (1978) Soziale Kompetenz. Experimentelle Ergebnisse zum Assertiveness-Training-Programm ATP. Meßmittel und Grundlagen, vol 1. Pfeiffer, München

Ullrich R, Ullrich de Muynck R, Peikert V, Crombach G (1975) Die Therapie multipler Situationsphobien (Platzangst) durch Habituationstraining (flooding) und periphere Erregungshemmung. Z Klin Psychol 4:209–233

Ullrich de Muynck R, Ullrich R (1976) Das Assertiveness-Training-Programm ATP: Einübung von Selbstvertrauen und sozialer Kompetenz. Pfeiffer, München

Ullrich de Muynck R, Ullrich R, Grawe K, Zimmer D (eds) (1980) Soziale Kompetenz. Experimentelle Ergebnisse zum Assertiveness-Training-Programm ATP. Klinische Effektivität und Wirkungsfaktoren, vol 2. Pfeiffer, München

Vollmer H, Kraemer S (eds) (1982) Ambulante Behandlung junger Alkoholabhängiger. Röttger, München

Wächter H-M, Pudel V (1980a) Kontrollierte Untersuchung einer extremen Kurzpsychotherapie (15 Stunden) mit dem Katathymen Bilderleben. Psychother Psychosom Med Psychol 30:193–205

Wächter H-M, Pudel V (1980b) Kurztherapie von 15 Sitzungen mit dem Katathymen Bilderleben. In: Leuner H (ed) Katathymes Bilderleben. Ergebnisse in Theorie und Praxis. Huber, Bern, pp 126–147

Westmeyer H (1976) Verhaltenstherapie: Anwendung von Verhaltenstheorien oder kontrollierte Praxis. In: Gottwald G, Kraiker C (eds) Zum Verhältnis von Theorie und Praxis in der Psychologie. Sonderheft I: 1976 der Mitteilungen der GVT. GVT, pp 3–37

Westmeyer H (1978) Wissenschaftstheoretische Grundlagen klinischer Psychologie. In: Baumann U, Berbalk H, Seidenstücker G (eds) Klinische Psychologie. Huber, Bern, pp 108–132 (Trends in Forschung und Praxis, vol 1)

Wittchen H-U, Fichter MM (1980) Psychotherapie in der Bundesrepublik. Beltz, Weinheim

Wittchen H-U, Fichter MM, Dvorak A, Zerssen D von (1980) Strukturelle Besonderheiten der psychotherapeutischen Versorgung. Psychotherapeuten und geographische Verteilung. Psychother Psychosom Med Psychol 30:95–107

Wittmann WW (1983) Evaluative Forschung in der Psychiatrie. In: Häfner H (ed) Forschung für die seelische Gesundheit. Springer, Berlin Heidelberg New York, pp 53–67

Wolfsteller HJ, Kächele H (1980) Behandlungserfahrungen im Rückblick. Eine Nachuntersuchung von 72 Patienten mit dem Struppschen Fragebogen. Unveröffentlichter Arbeitsbericht. Abteilung Psychotherapie, Universität Ulm

Zerssen D von (1979) Klinisch-psychiatrische Selbstbeurteilungs-Fragebögen. In: Baumann U, Berbalk H, Seidenstücker G (eds) Klinische Psychologie. Huber, Bern, pp 130–159 (Trends in Forschung und Praxis, vol 2)

Zerssen D von, Koeller D-M (1976) Klinische Selbstbeurteilungs-Skalen (KSb-S) aus dem Münchener Psychiatrischen Informations-System (PSYCHIS München). Manuale: Allgemeiner Teil; Die Beschwerden-Liste; Die Paranoid-Depressivitäts-Skala, sowie die Depressivitäts-Skala; Die Befindlichkeits-Skala. Beltz, Weinheim

Zerssen D von, Möller HJ (1980) Psychopathometrische Verfahren in der psychiatrischen Therapieforschung. In: Biefang S (ed) Evaluationsforschung in der Psychiatrie: Fragestellungen und Methoden. Enke, Stuttgart, pp 129–166

Zielke M (ed) (1982) Diagnostik in der Psychotherapie. Kohlhammer, Stuttgart

Overall Review of Research Strategies in Psychological Treatments in the French-Speaking Literature

E. A. SAND[1] and C. DE JONGHE

Introduction

At first sight, a division between the scientific literature written in English and that written in French seems arbitrary. We shall try to indicate to what extent, however, it is useful to identify the french-written research works as a separate entity.

In this presentation we will consider only books and articles concerning epidemiological or sociological research. Publications on clinical cases will not be analysed in spite of their interest. We also intend to examine only data about treatments used with adults. One should note the relative scarcity of books and articles written in French. The recent book of Gérin (1984), for example, quotes eight references to articles written in french in all list of two hundred.

Three kinds of approaches will be presented. The first part refers to general considerations, of a sociological or epistemological order, of research concerning psychological treatment. The second part presents investigations about methodological problems as seen by French speaking authors. Finally, the third part refers to the study of the effects of treatments, essentially estimates of the outcome, less frequently of the ongoing processes.

General Methodology of Research – Epistemological Aspects

Current medical experience, whether clinical or in the public health field, frequently encounters dilemmas that will, no doubt, be mentioned more than once during this meeting.

It is particularly difficult to combine research approaches which are fundamentally different, but which should, if possible, enrich one another. The clinical approach gathers a large amount of information on a single patient or small groups of patients. It takes account of individual "careers" starting, for example, the first contact with the therapist, during therapy and after it (follow-up). Even the grouping of a set of clinical observations may be difficult,

[1] Laboratoire d'Epidémiologie et de Médecine Sociale, Ecole de Santé Publique, Université Libre de Bruxelles, Campus Erasme, Route de Lennick 808, B-1070 Bruxelles

Psychological Treatment of Mental Illness
Edited by R. J. Daly and E. A. Sand

due to the large diversity of patients' characteristics. Epidemiological analysis, on the other hand, that will be of interest in public health, will often be based on slightly altered or simplified clinical data in order to offer a synthetic description of samples of patients.

Besides these obvious complexities and this paradox, it is clear that the personality of the therapist also intervenes in a determinant way (Benoit 1979; Paroden 1981). One can recall, by the way, the ideas of earlier psychotherapists, those of Freud of course, of Sacha Nacht (1950), etc. Bovet (1976) has indicated that research still remains at the stage of hypotheses, and that, among other factors, the multivariate character of the patient's and the therapist's personalities and their interaction set various problems. Nowadays, clinicians such as Rogers take an interest in the phenomenon of "empathy", i.e., "the capacity of understanding others emotionally" (Garrone 1981).

Bovet formulated some methodological indications. He insisted on the need to elaborate communicable indicators that might be transferred from one investigator or team to another. Four levels of analysis should be mentioned:

1. The analysis of the content *sensu stricto*
2. The analysis of the style
3. The analysis of the semantic differentiation tools (e.g. Osgood's scale)
4. The importance of avoiding interference of the observers.

Recently, Paul Gérin (1984) published a book on the evaluation of psychotherapies. He mentioned many important references (200), mostly written in English as mentioned before. He emphasized the need for clarification at various levels, starting with the general principles and the aims of the investigations as well as the disturbances caused to the studied phenomenon by the research itself. Gérin wrote that one should not forget the real dangers connected with "myths," defence reactions against anxiety, etc. He noted that these myths may, among other things, give rise to the temptation to take a very global approach to research, as opposed to a more restricted scientific approach, a more modest one that involves precise formulations of questions.

Gérin insisted on the need of codifying subjective elements, a difficult task indeed! The "captors" of the information may be the psychotherapist, the patient or an outside observer. The use of observation scales may also be useful, and it is important to make a judicious choice in this field. It is also important to determine clearly what kind of effects one intends to evaluate, or, as Gérin (1984, p. 54) stated, "what kind of patient, together with what kind of therapists will have a tendency to present what kind of effects or profile of modifications"? (see Abell and Wallot 1981, p. 1155).

Other authors, Chanoit et al. (1983) for example, have also emphasized these difficulties, together with the difficulty of reducing the role played by the personality of the therapist and by the patients' individuality. Chanoit quoted Robert Castel (1982) who remarks, as he has done often in his epistemological studies, that the function (of the psychotherapist) is to "find back, beyond the pathological episode, the meaning of an individual path (*trajectoire indivi-*

duelle) with regard to the history of the subject, or the meaning of his inscription in the social environment".

This return to the study of the individual is quite characteristic of the present scientific literature on methodology. In his recent work on the subject (*La place du désordre*), Boudon (1984) indicated to what extent the structures become obvious by starting with the individual actors and not taking a global approach.

This is how one progressively reaches an approach that is at the same time more accurate from the technical point of view and that also refers to a wider and more global system than the patient himself. Several authors, including Chanoit, have quoted an english-speaking author, Karasu (1982), who proposed four basic postulates and then defined what one could call a new paradigm. On the one hand, he emphasized the fact that psychotherapy is a communication process, a "dynamic field" that must be analysed. On the other hand, the research itself is also an interactive communication phenomenon (meta-communication). The context in which this communication takes place is obviously important. Finally, the object of investigation, of evaluation, is thus a real system of interactions between all these actors. It is in fact not an

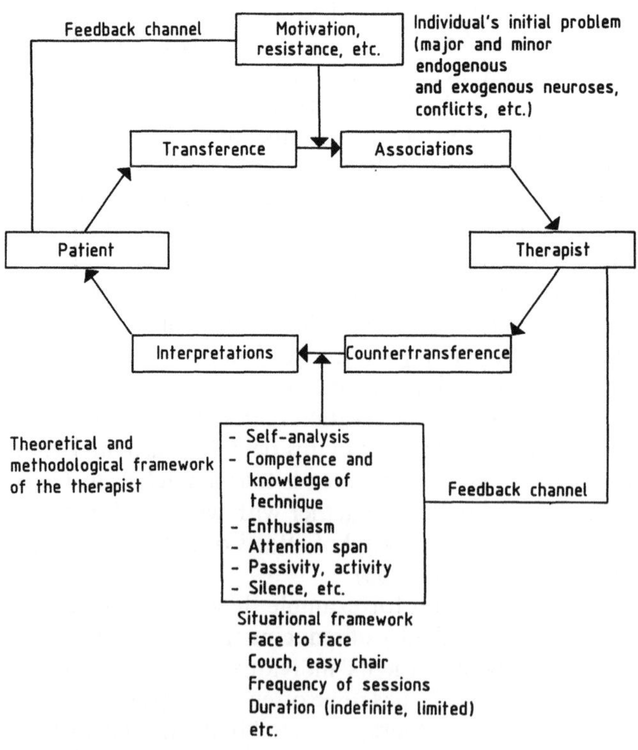

Fig. 1. Patient-therapist interaction (Translated from Gilliéron 1983)

experimental context, but a "real" one, (Benoit 1979; Hermann and Hovaguimian 1983).

We should note that some authors, Marchand and Crombez (1983) for example, think that one should widen the field of observation and in particular include the care unit in which the interaction occurs, if not the institution or even the psychiatric sector. The importance of the interaction between the patient and the therapist is also emphasized by Gilliéron (1983) who referred on this subject to the works of Malan. In order to clarify the significance of these propositions, Gilléron formulated an interesting scheme, shown in Fig. 1. This scheme indicates the chain of communication elements between the patient and the therapist, several mechanisms that act at the level of the patient, and also the means of control used by the therapist, or which he can at least consider. It is important to emphasize the role of the patient's motivation on the one hand and of the "enthusiasm" of the therapist on the other. The broader frame within which this relation occurs is important, whether it is "face to face" or a treatment on the couch. The role of the frequency of the sessions and of their duration must also not be neglected.

More generally, and no doubt in a way that differs from the one presented in the English and American literature, important authors insist on the necessity of considering the evaluation within its global context. Such an approach is full of difficulties or traps. However, it avoids neglecting the field of the relations between the various actors engaged in a psychological treatment. It also gives the opportunity to stress, as Robert Castel puts it "the influence of the individuality of these actors."

The majority of the authors who underline the difficulties arising from these approaches use terms like "impossible research," "undiscoverable witness," etc. Apart from clinical approaches, little if any evaluation research corresponding to these propositions has been carried out up to now.

One could gain the impression that the theoretical, epistemological, methodological requirements make it difficult to study "the arena of realities" the "game" that links therapist and patient, including their social environment. Fortunately, things that may be difficult from a theoretical point of view are not necessarily impossible in practice, as authors like Chanoit et al. (1983) have mentioned.

Applied Methodological Considerations

We endorse the assertion that what may be difficult to achieve in theory, can be achieved or at least approached in practice. Several authors have developed what one may call intervention patterns (*grilles d'intervention*) by means of which they have tried to systematize or catalogue, in a logical, exhaustive and precise way, interventions or relational phenomena occurring between the therapist and client (Aubert and Lalive 1978 a–c; Gilliéron 1983). For example, Aubert and Lalive (1978 a–c) presented an "attempt to analyze the psychotherapeutic conversations in ambulatory psychotherapy." The authors worked on so-called support treatments (*traitements de soutien*) and on the basis of the interactions observed between the interventions of the patient and of the therapist, elaborated a bidimensional analytic pattern. One of the dimensions refers to the interventions of the therapist and the other to the level or typology of these interventions: emission, recovery (*reprise*), and connection.

The authors recalled earlier studies by Barthes (1964), who defined several levels of manifestation concerning the patient: indication (*indice*), signal, image, and sign. Barthes defined those four levels as follows:

- Indication: no psychological representation – facts which are neither immediate nor existential
- Signal: no psychological representation – immediate and existentials facts
- Image: psychological representation – analogy, metaphore, or inadequate
- Sign: psychological representation – groundless or correct (corresponds to the *„décantation"* of a situation and to relational phenomena)

Taking into account observations on the patient, Aubert and Lalive considered various psychological approaches or interventions available to the therapist. These occur at the level of the "reality of the facts," i.e. of the "psychological universe," of the relations as already mentioned. The classification of these sets of elements, one concerning the patient, the other the therapist, leads to a pattern of exchanges relating the two systems, that allows the comparison, within an ongoing process, of various successive therapeutic sessions. These approaches may seem somewhat complex but the authors think it is possible to put them into practice.

Gérin et al. (1983) emphasized the interest of investigations carried out jointly in different centres, e.g. with the use of scales. They suggested the use of "modules" that can be applied in any centre (common work module) and other modules that can be optional or personalized and would only be used in one or several centres but not in all of them. It is clear that research projects of that kind, concerning a larger number of patients, are of great interest. Their complexity, however, must be considered.

As a synthesis of the presentation of these technical approaches, let us emphasize the fact that a great many of them concern the processes entered into during the psychological treatments and that they go beyond the observation or recording of the outcome, of the results observed at the end of the interventions. These approaches are going to a deeper level of analysis. This offers the advantage of not removing the subtleties and the dynamic aspects of the communication between therapist and client. However, it is impossible to deny the great difficulty of the application to an actual research project. This has, however, been realised by authors like Hermann and Hovaguimian (1983) who state that beyond the differences of the level of the "doctrines," common ways or modalities of intervention do exist in the various methods of psychotherapy.

Study of the Effects of Treatment

After the analysis of methodological issues and taking account of the difficulties that have been mentioned, we will present some examples of evaluations of outcome of psychological treatments. They were carried out on large enough samples of subjects to outweigh the purely clinical approach. We will first discuss a well known scale, that of Osgood, standardized mainly for Switzerland by Gilliéron and Bovet. It allows the evaluation of intrapsychic changes of patients. It is possible, according to the authors, to confirm or even to complete by means of this scale the clinical impressions gained by the therapists. It is a fact that the pattern seems to change during certain psychical treatments. It is not clear, however, whether this change corresponds to a real mobilization of intrapsychic mechanisms.

An interesting in-depth study was presented by Gilliéron (1983) in his book on short analytic psychotherapies. It is probably true, as the author emphasizes in agreement with other works on the subject, that short psychotherapy, because of its rather more precise character and the constraints that it imposes, allows one to achieve better evaluative approaches.

Gilliéron et al. (1980), in a catamnestic study of patients engaged in psychotherapy in Lausanne (1974–1976), used a questionnaire developed by the team that consisted of 29 questions. They concerned the troubles undergone by the patients, the reactions to these troubles, the relations between the patients and their social environment, the changes that occurred in these relations, and the opinion of the patients about the treatment factors that contributed to the observed change during the treatment, etc. This questionnaire also concerned other fields, but it is impossible to mention them all here. Forty questionnaires were sent to a group of general practitioners. Thirty-two questionnaires were finally considered and analysed by the team. The authors reported that they had no "pretension to put in evidence a deep structural change." The questionnaires were given to three different judges for the evaluation of the possible evolution.

Each judge had no knowledge of the opinions of the other judges before the end of the investigation. The task of the judges was to determine the "indications of improvement on the somato-psychical and relational level and in insight." The scale used had five levels: 0, worsening; 1, without change; 2, slight improvement; 3, average improvement; 4, good improvement; and 5, recovery. Each judge noted the possible improvement of somatic and psychic symptoms, of relational symptoms and the possible improvement in insight.

Figure 2 gives the distribution of scores from the three judges. The distributions differ slightly but the authors nevertheless were astonished by the good concordance of the judgments. Moreover, they calculated the inter-judge correlations that appeared to be significant: eight were highly significant ($P<0.001$), and one was significant at the level $P<0.01$. One may conclude that an inquiry of this kind proves the possibility of evaluating, in a quite ob-

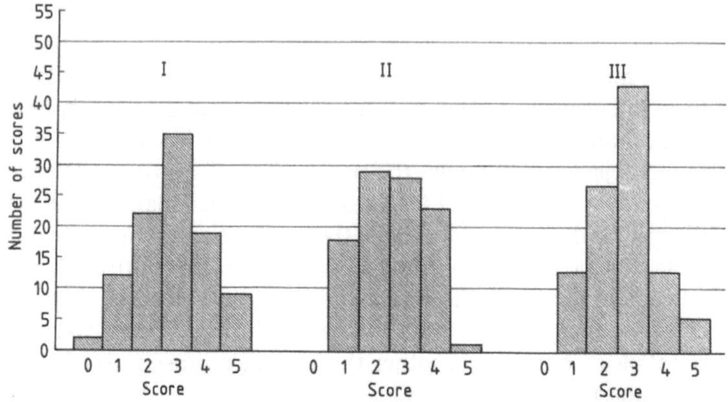

Fig. 2. Histogram of the scores given by the judges in the study of Gilliéron et al. (1980). Only the total scores (somatic and psychic symptoms, relational symptoms, insight) are given

jective way, the outcome of short-term psychotherapies using codified data, i.e. information about the evolution of particular signs or symptoms.

Gilliéron et al. (1980) emphasized in their conclusions the real interest of investigations of this type. One should stress that it is necessary that the temporal frame of a short psychotherapy be fixed from the beginning. Such therapies are more often brought to a successful conclusion. In contrast, vague indications, frequently if not in all cases, lead to failures and ruptures. And, finally the quality of the training and the experience of the psychotherapist are important elements for favourable progress and outcome. Moreover, this quality can be evaluated in different ways.

Conclusions

The examination, within a synoptic approach, of the studies and research that we have mentioned leads to a certain perplexity. Indeed, for well justified reasons a large number of studies put the reader on guard against research projects that are focused on too restricted a concept of the relational phenomenon called psychotherapy. We should recall on this subject the epistemological considerations quoted at the beginning.

At the same time, for similar reasons, authors like Castel (1982) or on a broader level Boudon (1984), warn against condensing in a model such highly complex psychological or social facts as, for example, the "path" (*trajectoire*) of a patient. Nevertheless, the main studies that have actually been carried out, studies that yield interesting conclusions and will probably lead to further progress in this field, go the opposite way and analyse limited aspects of psychological treatments. Moreover, whilst most French-speaking authors insist on the necessity of investigating the "process" involved in the dynamic of a psychotherapy, for the time being more research projects have been undertaken and mentioned in the French-speaking literature, which are limited to the narrower but more precise field of "outcome"!

Those who may want to carry out a project in this field are confronted by contradictory messages. One may even consider, hence the perplexity, that the situation looks like a "mission impossible." As a matter of fact, in various other fields of research on social and psychosocial issues, numbers of different methods have been developed which may not be, for the time being, combined or integrated. This is simply due to the complexity of the fields of investigation and to their multidimensional character. Contradictions of this kind, whether apparent or real, will probably persist for some time.

The pendulum movement will go on between the extremes. On one side are the epidemiological methods, based on numerical data, statistical analysis, and concerning rather clearly defined and if possible important samples. On the other side are studies carried out, often on smaller samples, using more comprehensive kinds of information such as the personality of the patient and the therapist, possibly their social environment, and the "process" of the treatment.

One can expect that in the not too distant future, because of the rapid progress of the data-analysis methods, the more clinically oriented, comprehensive approaches and the epidemiological methods will come closer and finally complement and enrich each other.

References

Abel T, Wallot H (1981) Recherche évaluative et psychiatrie. L'Information Psychiatrique 57:1145–1162

Aubert C, Lalive J (1978a) Essai d'analyse des entretiens psychothérapiques en psychiatrie ambulatoire. I. Les interventions du psychothérapeute. Psychologie Médicale 10:1515–1521

Aubert C, Lalive J (1978b) Essai d'analyse des entretiens psychothérapieques en psychiatrie ambulatoire. II. Les propos du patient. Psychologie Médicale 10:1525–1530

Aubert C, Lalive J (1978c) Essai d'analyse des entretiens psychothérapiques en psychiatrie ambulatoire. III. Grilles d'analyse sémiologique des entretiens psychothérapiques. Psychologie Médicale 10:1533–1540

Barthes R (1964) Le degré zéro de l'écriture. Eléments de sémiologie. Gonthier, Paris

Benoit J (1979) Modèles d'interaction et d'intervention en psychothérapie. Psychologie Médicale 11:351–356

Boudon R (1984) La place du désordre. Presse Universitaire de France, Paris

Bovet J (1976) Effets des psychothérapies et évaluations. In: Schneider P (ed) Propédeutique d'une psychothérapie. Payot, Paris

Castel R (1982) La gestion des risques. Editions de Minuit, Paris

Chanoit PF, Sideris N, De Barsy D, Gaubert B, Cohen S (1983) Les pièges de l'évaluation dans les traitements psychologiques. Annales Médico-Psychologiques 141:606–611

Garrone G (1981) Les psychothérapies. Etat actuel et perspectives. Archives Suisses Neurologiques 120:197–210

Gérin P (1984) L'évaluation des psychothérapies. Presse Universitaire de France, Paris

Gérin P, Widlocher D, Sali A, Hanauer MT, Baguet J (1983) Possibilité et intérêt d'enquêtes multicentriques pour l'évaluation des psychothérapies. Annales Médico-Psychologiques 141:620–633

Gilliéron E, Merceron C, Piolino P, Rossel F (1980) L'évaluation des psychothérapies analytiques brèves et de longue durée: comparaison et devenir. Psychologie Médicale 12:623–637

Gilliéron E (1983) Aux confins de la psychoanalyse (psychothérapies analytiques brèves, acquisitions actuelles). Payot, Paris

Hermann, P, Hovaguimian T (1983) Une méthode d'évaluation des interventions du thérapeute dans le cadre d'entretiens a visée psychothérapique. Annales Médico-Psychologiques 141:601–605

Karasu TB (1982) Proving the efficiency of psychotherapy to government: A bureaucratic solution? Am J Psychiatry 139 (Editorial)

Marchand P, Crombez Y (1983) Regards sur la valeur des psychothérapies au sein du „complexe" service-secteur. Annales Médico-Psychologiques 141:622–626

Nacht S (1950) De la pratique à la théorie psychoanalytique. Presse Universitaire de France, Paris

Pardoen D (1981) Les données actuelles de la recherche en psychothérapie. Acta Psychiatrica Belgica 81:521–531

Efficacy of Psychological Treatments for Mental Illness: A Review of Papers in the English Language

R. J. DALY[1] and H. A. ROSS

Introduction

Doctors have always been eager to see their personal interactions with their patients as being part of the art of medicine. Until the time of Freud they were extremely reluctant to examine critically the nature of these interactions and their effects on the course of illnesses of their patients. There has, however, been increasing interest in examining the possibilities for applying the methodological rigour previously only used in physical treatments, to psychological treatments. This workshop concerns itself with pointing to needs for further research. In earlier papers I have reviewed the problems concerning research on the effectiveness of psychotherapy in general (Daly 1983), and for psychoses in particular (Daly 1984).

This review of the literature concerning efficacy of psychological treatment is confined mostly to work published since the mid- 1970s. However, a few important earlier papers are included. Glass (1984) reviewed the situation optimistically. He pointed to the problem of the outcome influencing process in this area of research. Aspects of therapy usually considered as independent variables influence outcome (e.g. therapeutic climate and specific actions by the patient or therapist), and may also be affected by the emerging outcome of the treatment. Thus, the "variables" may be consequences of outcome rather than causes. He pointed out that psychotherapies are not readily reproducible "technologies" but are treatments composed of many detailed parts with a continuously changing set of interactions between therapists and patients. Nevertheless, he pointed to the increasing reliance on empirical studies based on scientific methodology rather than untested presuppositions. He felt that the evaluation of the competence and skill of psychotherapists was an area requiring further evaluation, but pointed to the continuing difficulty of assessing how various levels of the clinical process affect outcome for specific patients.

Prioleau et al. (1983) challenged the work of Glass and his colleagues in their meta-analysis mentioned below. By confining themselves to studies that contained a psychotherapy and a placebo treatment they concluded that for real patients (as opposed to volunteers) there was no evidence that the benefits of psychotherapy were greater than those for placebo treatment.

[1] University Department of Psychiatry, Cork Regional Hospital, Wilton, Cork, Ireland

Psychological Treatment of Mental Illness
Edited by R. J. Daly and E. A. Sand

The study of Prioleau et al. (1983) was quoted in an editorial in the *British Medical Journal* in March 1984, by Michael Shepherd. He pointed out that some of the obstacles to research in this area can be overcome. Nevertheless, he noted that most of the major research bodies in the United Kingdom appeared to fight shy of the topic and that professional organizations, including the Royal College of Psychiatrists, have done little more than pay lip-service to the need for action. In general he supported the conclusion of Prioleau et al. and quoted Jerome Frank: "whith many patients the placebo may be as effective as psychotherapy because the placebo condition contains the necessary, and possibly the sufficient, ingredient for much of the beneficial effect of all forms of psychotherapy. This is a helping person who listens to the patients' complaints and offers a procedure to relieve them, thereby inspiring the patients' hopes in combating demoralisation." Shepherd's view as outlined in this editorial is not unusual in Europe: "an undefined technique applied to unspecified cases with unpredictable results. For this technique rigorous training is required."

The aim of this review is to discover how effective psychotherapy had been seen to be by a wide range of people in the field, and also how the task of establishing efficacy was tackled. Approximately half of the reviewed articles involve some kind of experimental research while the other half are reviews or discussions.

Disorders

Neurotic Disorders

The vast majority of the target illnesses of psychotherapy are neurotic disorders, as these patients have unimpaired reality testing and consequently remain relatively more receptive than psychotics.

Andrews and Harvey (1982) reanalysed the data of Smith et al. (1980) to answer the question "Does psychotherapy benefit neurotic patients?" Only studies concerning neurosis (of which there are 81) were used in their meta-analysis. They found that psychotherapy was effective and claimed that "the condition of the typical patient after treatment was better than that of 77% of untreated controls measured at the same time." Andrews and Harvey (1982) also noted that behavioural and psychodynamic verbal therapies were superior to all others. Follow-up showed the improvement to be maintained for up to at least a year.

Bovill (1977) studied the efficacy of group psychotherapy with a psychoanalytic orientation and the use of behavioural techniques and relaxation on 72 neurotic patients. Of the original 36 patients in each of the treated and control groups, only 30 of the former and 24 of the latter could later be traced. The measure of success was the inverse of days spent hospitalized. Although the treated group improved significantly more, the control group also im-

Table 1. The findings of Ellis (1957)

Type of therapy (no. of patients)	"Little or no improvement"		"Distinct improvement"		"Considerable improvement"	
	%	*n*	%	*n*	%	*n*
Psychoanalysis (16)	50	8	37	6	13	2
Psychoanalytically oriented (78)	37	29	45	35	18	14
Rational (78)	10	8	46	36	44	34

proved in the interim period, and as regards days spent in hospital, spent only one-third of the expected time there. They had anticipated this to some extent from knowledge of the spontaneous remission rate. Bovill's findings were that this type of therapy was not only an effective treatment, but also an economical one from the point of view of therapists' time.

Ellis, in 1957, employed three techniques of psychotherapy on both neurotic and a few borderline psychotic patients. The three techniques were psychoanalytic psychotherapy, psychoanalytically oriented psychotherapy and rational therapy. This latter is directed at showing the patient how his current beliefs are illogical and groundless; the patient is made to review his underlying philosophies and is taught to think "straight." Rational psychotherapy is not unlike cognitive therapy in its restructuring techniques. Table 1 shows that rational therapy produced the greatest number of people who improved considerably, while psychoanalysis produced the least. However, Ellis was cautious in interpreting his results, and noted certain characteristics of the successful patients such as intelligence, willingness to work and acceptance of the therapist's directions. No account was taken of the spontaneous remission rate by use of a control group.

A third study, by Lazarus (1963), involved 126 cases of severe neurosis which were treated with behavioural therapy. Lazarus split the disorders into 12 categories so that he could assess the improvement in a more structured way. Of the 126 cases, 78 (61.9%) were rated as "markedly improved," and these improvements were found to last throughout treatment and the follow-up of a mean of 2.15 years. Again, however, no account was taken of a spontaneous remission rate by use of a control group.

Segraves and Smith (1976) only looked at three cases of neurosis while investigating the feasibility of treating patients with two different kinds of therapies simultaneously. Psychoanalytically orientated therapy and behaviour therapy were the two treatments involved. The involvement took the form of a referral from the former to the latter therapy for attention to a specific symptom. The linked-therapy approach was deemed to be a success and expected pitfalls, such as the patient playing one therapist off against the other or withdrawing from the analytic therapy once the symptom removal was achieved, did not occur. Segraves and Smith described the experiments accurately as a pilot study and suggested that they produced encouragement for further research.

In the next section more specific illness such as anxiety, phobias and depression are covered.

Anxiety

There are four separate but connected articles by Hans Strupp (1980 a–d) where the main illness is anxiety, (accompanied by depression and social withdrawal). For each article two cases were drawn for comparison from the Vanderbilt psychotherapy project (Strupp and Hadley 1979), whose primary aim was "to investigate the relative contribution of a therapist's technical skills and the qualities inherent in any good human relationship to outcome in time-limited psychotherapy." Their main hypothesis was not supported, i.e. that given a benign human relationship technical skills of professional psychotherapists did not produce a greater therapeutic change than did the ordinary supportive skills of the college professors, i.e. laymen. All patients improved and maintained an improvement at the follow-up a year later. Strupp and Hadley pointed out that the therapy was time limited, and that the subjects were young and changeable, and only midly disturbed.

The first article by Strupp began the systematic comparisons with a pair of patients, one who succeeded in therapy and one who failed. The comparison stressed the importance of patient variables as factors determining outcome in time-limited psychotherapy. In this study the patient variables for success appeared to be maturity, admission and acceptance of the existence of a problem, and motivation to seek help and to work for resolution of the problem. Strupp recommended, as far as is possible, adapting the therapeutic techniques to the patient, and not the other way around.

The second article of this series followed a very similar format, and indeed produced the same conclusion with regard to patient variables. The patient who was deemed a therapeutic failure was characterised by a lack of motivation, a negative and even hostile attitude, immaturity and constant denial of the existence of problems. Strupp's third article took on a new variable, that of the performance of a lay counsellor. Again, two cases of male college students showing anxiety were compared, one a success, the other a failure. The important finding of the study was that "fundamental differences do exist between a trained and an untrained therapist's approach to psychotherapy." The difficulties the counsellor had with the failed patient involved a lack of training, although it was unclear whether this was a cause or an effect. The patient's awareness of the therapist's level of training highlights the problem of control and objectivity in this kind of research. Strupp defined the difference between two therapists as qualitative and therefore very difficult to measure.

The final article of this quartet reaffirmed the findings of the other three. An experienced psychotherapist was employed and felt that the greatest problem with the failed patient was his being pushed into therapy by outside agents rather than seeking it himself. Again, the need to cater to the patient, to the individual, was stressed and the suggestion was tendered that perhaps training alone does not make the therapist.

Phobias

With regard to psychological treatment of phobias, behaviour therapy in general, and hierarchial desensitization in particular, seem to be the treatments chosen most often. The explanation for this is of course, that the illness presents an easily identifiable symptom in which the problem manifests itself. Desensitization, the gradual exposing of the patient to the feared object or situation, therefore seems ideal. However, all four of the papers reviewed compared it with other therapies to see if it was indeed the best choice.

Gelder et al. (1967) compared desensitization with individual psychotherapy and group psychotherapy (psychoanalytically orientated). Sixteen subjects were allocated to each of desensitization and group therapy, but only 10 to individual psychotherapy (due to a lack of skilled therapists). The presenting complaint was a severe phobia, i.e. having at least a 4.1 rating on a 1–5 scale. The findings of this study were that desensitization was initially significantly better than group therapy and (not significantly) better than individual psychotherapy, but at termination had lost its advantage. Of the 62 patients, 17 were much improved, 20 improved and 25 unchanged, which means that between the three types of therapy only half the patients involved were helped. Desensitization did provide faster improvement as well as producing "more patients whose symptoms improved at the end of treatment and follow-up." Only two patients improved "completely," both with desensitization.

Gillan and Rachman (1974) aimed to replicate and extend the study of Gelder et al. (1967). They also sought to isolate the effects of various components of desensitization treatment and to collect data on the relationships between psychophysiological changes and clinical outcome. Their study involved four treatments. Pseudotherapy consisted of instruction in muscle relaxation and at no time did the phobia receive any direct focus. The systematic desensitization group were given basic treatment and presented with phobic stimuli while relaxed. The second desensitization group also received hierarchical desensitization, but the phobic items were presented without the patients being trained in relaxation techniques. The psychotherapy group were given a combination of individual, insight and rational therapy.

There was a total of 32 subjects, eight in each group. The treatment was fairly intensive with twice weekly sessions lasting from 45 to 60 minutes. The average duration of therapy was 3 months. A battery of tests, including ratings by patients, therapists and an independent assessor, personality and behaviour avoidance tests and psychophysiological assessments, was employed.

Desensitization, with or without relaxation, proved to be more successful than either pseudotherapy or psychotherapy at termination, but this finding had diminished at follow-up. Except in the area of psychotherapy, agreement between the patients, therapists and assessor on the ratings was strong. For psychotherapy therapists tended to rate the outcome more favourably than the others. Gillan and Rachman felt they had succeeded in their primary aim of replicating the study of Gelder et al. (1967).

A study of the treatments of phobias (Hussain, 1971) compared desensitization and flooding (implosion) in a controlled crossover trial. The 40 patients taking part had either agoraphobia or social phobias. Whereas desensitization is a gradual exposure of the patient to his fear, flooding consists of forcing the patient to remain in the presence of the feared stimulus while avoidance responses are prevented or blocked. The Pavlovian term is response prevention. Both therapies were assisted either by 20 ml 1.25% thiopental sodium or by 20 ml saline infusions applied intravenously.

The overall finding was that desensitization patients, regardless of whether thiopental or saline infusions were being given, continued to show progressive improvement. However, thiopental-assisted flooding proved to be the most successful treatment, as the amount of change per patient was more than 50% greater with this treatment than with desensitization and markedly greater than with saline-assisted flooding.

Behaviour therapy and supportive therapy were compared in another paper on the treatment of phobias by Klein et al. (1983), who divided an unspecified number of patients randomly between three groups: (1) behaviour therapy and imipramine hydrochloride, (2) behaviour therapy and a placebo, and (3) supportive therapy and imipramine.

The supportive therapy was dynamically orientated and non-directive. The behaviour therapy was described as relaxation training, systematic desensitization in imagination, homework assignments and assertiveness training. The patients in the behavioural therapy group also appeared to receive supportive therapy, given by the authors.

The results of the study, although not clearly described, showed no significant differences between the three diagnostic group (agoraphobia, mixed phobias and simple phobias). Most treatments brought about a high degree of improvement, but only one of 18 analyses found any difference between the two therapies and this was in favour of behavioural therapy.

The authors stated openly that they expected behavioural therapy to do better and considered the fact that the supportive therapy did well surprising. A large section of the discussion is devoted to explaining, and, to some extent, trying to discount this. In the only instance where behavioural therapy was found to be more effective, the authors admit to the possibility of bias by a non-blind therapist. Since the behavioural therapy was reported to include supportive therapy, the implications of the study are confusing.

Depression

Cognitive therapy has become an attractive option for depressed patients and has the appeal to the investigator of being readily susceptible to measurement.

Many of the papers reviewed here look at this type of therapy whether alone or in combination with another treatment.

Bari Koalta (1981), reporting on the National Institute of Mental Health's mega-trial of psychotherapies, focused on the fact that the study of depression was to take a large part in the trial because it is seen as a major public health problem. Twenty-five per cent of all Americans become depressed to the point of needing professional help at some point during their lives and depression is a leading cause of suicide. The need to study depression seriously and as a matter of some urgency is also underlined by the fact that it accounts for some 75% of all psychiatric hospitalizations in the United States.

Blackburn et al. (1981) treated 64 depressed patients with cognitive therapy, drugs and a combination of the two. This latter method proved to be superior to the individual methods both in hospital and in general practice. In general practice alone, cognitive therapy was superior to drug therapy. The authors commented in their discussion that the depression classification as it stands may be too broad.

Rush et al. (1977) showed that depressed patients improved to a greater degree with cognitive therapy than they did with imipramine pharmacotherapy, although these patients also improved significantly.

Hopelessness and self-concept specifically are the targets of another study by Rush et al. (1982). Although they did not cite Blackburn et al. (1981) the commendation made in the latter article that depression should be subclassified is followed through. Cognitive therapy again proved to be better than pharmacotherapy, with better results for hopelessness than self-concept which would therefore appear not be be an indication of depression.

Klerman et al. (1974) in their research sought ways of preventing relapse and they compared the efficacy of the tricyclic antidepressant amitriptyline with individual psychotherapy. One hundred and fifty depressed female patients were involved. The results showed a greater relapse rate for those on psychotherapy alone as opposed to those on amitriptyline with a little psychotherapy. Drug therapy with psychotherapy proved not to be significantly different from psychotherapy alone, but psychotherapy was seen to be beneficial with problems of social adjustment and interpersonal relationships.

Rounsaville et al. (1981) asked different questions in their article on whether psychotherapy and pharmacotherapy for depression conflict. Psychotherapy and pharmacotherapy are often used in combination as treatment for depressive patients. But Rounsaville et al. (1981) sought to answer speculations that had been cast on the positive or benign effect it had been said to produce. About 56 patients took part in the final trial. Pharmacotherapy with psychotherapy and psychotherapy alone were tested, with six hypotheses formulated to discover if any negative effects of either therapy on the other were present. None of the six hypotheses were supported by the data and the findings were, as with other studies, that a combination of the two methods not only does not produce negative effects, but proves superior to either treatment alone.

Weissman (1979) reviewed 17 clinical trials that tested psychological treatments for depression. Her overall conclusion was that psychotherapy is better than no treatment, and is as good as but no better than drugs. A combination method is therefore the most efficacious, with drugs affecting symptoms and psychotherapy affecting social functioning.

These three studies have shown then that cognitive therapy is an effective treatment for depression and leads to a very good symptomatic response.

In my previous review of the efficacy of psychotherapy for psychoses I pointed out that while the feeling has grown up that psychotherapy in psychotic patients has negligible or even harmful effects, the costs of paying personnel in mental hospitals exceeds the bill for medications by a very large factor. This surely provides justification for examining what these expensive personnel do and say during their encounters with schizophrenic patients.

Schizophrenia

Psychotherapy does not appear to be the treatment of choice for psychotic patients, as in many cases a lack of contact with reality is a prevalent feature of the illness. Drugs must be used to control this symptom in particular and to help establish communication in general with the patient. However, six papers herein reviewed dealt with psychotherapy and schizophrenic patients.

Beck et al. (1981) looked at 35 schizophrenics and their therapists in comparison with 20 patients who were not in long-term psychotherapy. Psychotherapy patients were found to differ from the others by class, marital status and isolation. Schizophrenics in therapy were of a higher social class. They were, in fact, failures in the sense that independently functioning schizophrenics did not attend psychotherapy: "These patients are typically not those who make substantial improvements."

Leff et al. (1982) employed social intervention with the families of schizophrenic patients, all of whom were maintained on neuroleptic drugs. This kind of intervention was aimed at reducing overinvolvement, usually of a parent or sibling, increasing or decreasing contact levels as desired, and as an information source. The therapy was deemed to be a success as relapses were far less frequent in these cases than in the control group.

O'Brien et al. (1972) compared group psychotherapy with individual psychotherapy as treatments for 100 schizophrenic out patients. Outcome scores based on social functioning and psychiatric ratings for the group therapy patients were found to be significantly better than those in individual therapy, although rehospitalization rates did not differ significantly. The absence of a control group in this study is a flaw.

These three studies then did not display an overwhelming enthusiasm for psychotherapy as a treatment for schizophrenia, although the tendency was to see it as beneficial rather than non-effective or harmful, at least in a context of providing factual information and therefore better understanding of the illness to patients and their families.

The other papers were reviews of literature, research and psychotherapy. The latter was found in a chapter by Gwynne Jones (1978) in the book *Schizophrenia: Towards a New Synthesis*. The author touches on psychotherapy, (i.e. psychodynamic therapies) and says "supportive therapy in general is necessary as it is in all psychiatric illnesses, but that psychoanalysis has not been shown to be a success in this area." Family therapy is of value, however, especially with younger, acute schizophrenics at home. Again, family therapy, like social intervention, is group therapy for the family which provides a forum for the direct release of feelings and emotions so that together the unit may work more closely with greater understanding of the problem.

Under individual therapies, Gwynne Jones takes a passing but well deserved look at the relatively new personal construct therapy which was formulated by Bannister (1983) from Kelly's original theory (1955). There is little research available on this topic to date and still less positive findings but it is nevertheless favourably reviewed. Personal construct therapy involves long-term serial validation to tighten weak construing. Non-psychotic people are consistent in their constructs, but patients suffering from thought disorder are not. Therefore, it is to this specific problem that construct psychotherapists attend.

Behaviour therapy is dealt with in great detail. Gwynne Jones distinguishes between behaviour therapy per se and behaviour modification which is the operant conditioning paradigm of Skinner. This involves studying behaviour patterns and reinforcing the desirable factors while ignoring the less desirable ones. Often the therapist instructs parents or teachers in the appropriate techniques, as behaviour modification is most effective in the patient's own environment.

Gwynne Jones cites Ullman and Krasner (1969) who "suggest that schizophrenic behaviour is the result of repeated failure of reinforcement or certain sequences of behaviour from which the schizophrenic patient learns not to attend to the usual environmental cues related to reinforcement especially the social stimuli to which normal people respond." Although these theories have not been proven many therapists who use operant conditioning accept them, and as operant techniques have been successful in changing the behaviour of schizophrenic patients, they take this as their justification.

Gwynne Jones explores the idea of token economies introduced by Ayllon and Azrin (1968) and says that the evidence of the success of the system is strong.

In a chapter in the *Comprehensive Textbook of Pschiatry* May (1980) commended the review of Luborsky et al. (1980) of psychotherapy outcome, but faulted it for failing to distinguish between schizophrenic and non-schizophrenia patients as subjects. There is, he claimed, a great difference in the effect psychotherapy can have between the two groups. He divided the group up again into inpatients and outpatients and re-reviewed personal studies in this new context.

For inpatients, seven individual psychotherapy studies provided May with the basic conclusion that psychotherapy did no good at all, especially if the schizophrenic patient was so bad as to be hospitalized. Fourteen standard group-therapy papers also produced an overall negative result. The controls regarding medication were rather weak in nine further studies of other types of group therapy, making the outcome there of "weakly positive" rather suspect.

With outpatients three individual psychotherapy studies showed that psychotherapy is effective when used in conjunction with drugs, but noted adverse effects on withdrawn patients. Group therapy was found to be better than no therapy or individual therapy in five studies. Under the heading "Psychotherapy and Drugs," summaries of 36 relevant studies are presented.

McGlashan's paper in 1982 was on DSM III schizophrenia, and individual psychotherapy. McGlashan listed and described the five categories schizophrenia is now defined by, and explored them by means of recommending either supportive psychotherapy or investigative psychotherapy or both for each case.

Epstein and Vlok (1981) reviewed a number of "well designed" studies on the effect of psychotherapy on schizophrenia. The first study they reviewed was by May et al., who undertook a study of no less than five different methods of treatment over 2–5 years. The five therapies were individual psychotherapy alone, ataraxic drugs alone, individual psychotherapy and ataraxic drugs, electroconvulsive therapy, (ECT) and milieu treatment. The measure of success was the length of stay in hospital and on this measure the psychotherapy-alone group did least well; the milieu therapy group did a little better, while patients receiving ECT, drugs alone or psychotherapy plus drugs stayed in hospital for a far shorter time.

The study of May et al. concluded that drugs alone should be the preferred treatment for schizophrenia. However, they dismissed another finding from their own study; that the psychotherapy plus drugs group did slightly better than the drugs-alone group. Their more publicized finding has influenced some to dismiss the possibility of treating schizophrenic patients by psychotherapy at all, whereas there are in fact several indications that psychotherapy has been much underrated in this area.

Epstein and Vlok (1981) also commented on a review by May, who found group therapy, focused on reality or on a group activity, to be the most effective psychotherapy for schizophrenic patients. This is also true for the less frequent outpatient psychotherapy studies which have been done. The optimal orientation of therapy is to support and rehabilitation rather than to the ideal of promoting insight. Antipsychotic drug therapy is still the most effective treatment, though psychotherapy can play a role in improving social and occupational skills.

Hogarty and Goldberg (1973) commented on a study of a 2-year post-hospital treatment of 374 schizophrenic patients. The initial treatment was major role therapy (social case work and vocational rehabilitation) and chlorpromazine. After 2 months, patients were either assigned to drug or placebo groups. The overall results of the three papers written from this study were that major role therapy had no significant effects. However, only 48% of drug-treated patients relapsed compared with 80% of placebo-treated patients. Drug treatment was significantly more effective for women than men. The three papers note that major role therapy can have an adverse effect, i.e. cause a relapse in patients with severe symptoms.

Schooler (1978) compared psychological treatments with drugs and found that in the areas where drugs were least effective, psychotherapy was most beneficial. Specific behaviours should be the goals and not general personality change. Vaughn and Leff looked at the effects on families and found that those patients with relatives who have "low expressed emotions" were less likely to be rehospitalized.

Treatment

Psychodynamic Therapies

Psychoanalytic treatment, the oldest of the four main schools of psychotherapy, tries to unravel internal problems by bringing the unconscious neurotic conflict into the patient's conscious. Symptoms are not the target, but the underlying cause of them is. The formula for exploring the unconscious depths is to clarify confront and interpret. The therapist–patient relationship is used for the emergence of repressed childhood conflicts.

Beck et al. (1981) investigated psychodynamic therapy with schizophrenic patients and found it to be of some use. However, the limitations were apparent as only a certain type of patient underwent therapy, i.e. those with impaired social functioning. Patients who were able to function independently did not remain in psychotherapy.

Burke et al. (1979) looked at short-term therapies and calls brief psychoanalytic psychotherapy, the interpretive approach (Malan 1976; Sifneos 1973). Here intelligent, motivated people are selected for an intensive course which can be anxiety provoking.

Ellis (1957) compared orthodox psychoanalysis, psychoanalytically orientated psychotherapy and rational therapy with neurotic and borderline patients. The psychoanalysis group fared least well; the analytically orientated group did a little better while the rational therapy group did much better. No control group was involved.

Eysenck (1952) in his controversial article stated that "patients treated by means of psychoanalysis improve to the extent of 44%, whereas patients treated eclectically improve to 64%, and patients treated only custodially or by general practitioners improve to 72%." He included drop-outs as failures and excluded all studies lacking proper controls.

Gwynne Jones (1978) stated that dynamic psychoanalytically orientated therapy was not generally considered to be useful in schizophrenia, noting the claim of Rogers et al. (1967) for some success in the area for client-centred (empathy orientated) therapy.

Luborsky et al. (1975) reviewed many studies and found few differences in results between types. Four dynamically orientated therapies, client-centred and other traditional therapies were compared but were found not to differ significantly.

Marmor (1971) discussed the compatability of dynamic and behavioural therapies and felt they were much alike.

Segraves and Smith (1976) attempted to combine psychoanalytically orientated therapy with behaviour therapy in three cases of neurosis and found the combination to be extremely successful.

Sloane et al. (1975) compared short-term analytically orientated psychotherapy, behaviour therapy and a control group. Although all three groups improved significantly, the two treated groups improved more than the waiting list group. There was no difference between the improvements of the two treated groups. The improvement was found to be maintained at 1-year and 2-year follow-ups.

Strupp (1980 a–d), outlined eight cases treated with time-limited psychoanalytic psychotherapy, four successes and four failures. The patient factors influencing success were believed to be maturity, intelligence, acceptance of a problem, motivation and preparedness to work for a successful resolution. Psychoanalysts, for the most part, have been unable to cope with Eysenck's challenge of 1952. As Luborsky et al. (1975) commented, very few studies have been done which are specifically designed to test the effectiveness of psychoanalysis as opposed to other therapies or control groups. They felt that the dynamic nature of the therapy is often abused by charismatic-type therapies and that the confrontation part of the formula is expounded relentlessly to the detriment of the whole discipline.

Behaviour Therapy

Most behaviour therapy derives from laboratory studies of learning processes. The problem is defined in terms of a specific behaviour that the patient or society considers maladaptive, rather than in terms of unconscious conflict. The aim of treatment is to change behaviour – to change specifically its frequency, intensity and appropriateness (Parloff 1976).

Andrews and Harvey (1981) in their reanalysis of Smith, Glass and Miller's data (1980) found behaviour therapy (and psychodynamic verbal therapies) to be superior to all other treatments.

Earll and Kincey (1982) looked at behaviour therapy versus no treatment with 42 or 50 referred patients for a period of 2 years. Among other measures, subjects' use of the National Health Service was monitored throughout treatment and follow-up. During treatment both groups received medication but the treated group received significantly less than the control group. However, this finding did not continue through follow-up. There was no statistically significant difference between the two groups on any other objective or subjective measure. It must be noted that the medication was administered by general practitioners and was not directed by the therapists.

Epstein and Vlok (1981) in their literature review cited Russell's (1974) comment that "in many areas of practical application, behaviour therapy has been found to be either not very effective or no more effective than almost any other treatment." He suggested initially that non- specific factors, especially placebo effects, account for a large proportion of the success of desensitization in particular, but later added that there was not enough evidence to prove this. Aversion therapy for autistic children he considered effective, however, and the preferred treatment in this area.

Gelder et al. (1967) found desensitization for phobic patients significantly superior to group therapy in a trial including individual therapy. At termination none of the three treatments was significantly better than any other, but desensitization did show faster improvement.

Gillan and Rachman (1974) compared desensitization (with and without relaxation training) to pseudo-therapy and psychotherapy (individual, insight and rational). Desensitization was found to be the most effective treatment at the termination of the study but this statistical significance did not continue at follow-up.

Gwynne Jones (1978) reviewed behaviour therapy in a chapter on psychological treatments of schizophrenic inpatients. Behaviour modification was seen as more relevant to schizophrenia than behaviour therapy per se. Behavioural group therapy was singled out as the most promising development, but the token economy (Ayllon and Azrin 1968) represented the major application of behaviour modification in this area to date.

In a study by Hussain (1971), desensitization and flooding were compared either when assisted by thiopental or saline infusions in 40 phobic patients. Desensitization patients improved more overall and thiopental-assisted desensitization patients improved the most, by far.

Klein et al. (1983) compared behaviour therapy and supportive psychotherapy in the treatment of phobic patients. All patients improved markedly, but no real differences were found between the effects of the two therapies.

Lazarus (1963) looked at the results of behaviour therapy alone on 126 of his own severe neurosis cases. He found that 61.9% markedly improved or completely recovered. Neither a control group nor objective ratings were employed.

Luborsky et al. (1975) reviewed and compared many studies including 19 behavioural therapy trials. In six of these behaviour therapy emerged as superior and in 12 as no different. Tied scores appeared to be the norm, but happily no study reported negative or adverse effects.

Marks (1976) in discussing the current status of behavioural psychotherapy commented that although it is "hardly a panacea for all ills, the behavioural approach is the treatment of choice for certain selected problems." These problems include phobic disorders, social anxieties, obsessive-compulsive rituals and some sexual dysfunctions or deviations. For children, behaviour therapy can help nocturnal enuresis and phobias. Behaviour therapy still needs to prove its efficacy in related areas such as habit disorders, appetitive disorders and conversion hysteria. Marks felt that areas where behaviour therapy was ineffective were acute schizophrenia, depression and hypomania.

Marmor (1971) discussed the common ground of behavioural therapy and dynamic psychotherapy and emphasized the importance of behaviour therapy in this field.

Weissman (1979) reviewed eight studies on the efficacy of behavioural therapy with depression, but of these only three were complete. In these three, behavioural therapy took the form of self-control or monitoring and proved more effective than no treatment, non-directive groups or social skills. Only one of the three studies contained a control group.

Parloff (1976) while "shopping for the right therapy" said of behavioural modification that it is "particularly useful in some specific classes of phobias, some forms of compulsive or ritual behaviour and some sexual dysfunctions." He also made reference to the speed of improvement in areas like addiction, alcoholism and smoking but added that these types of improvements usually do not last. Parloff's conclusions appear to be an adequate summary of the efficacy of behavioural therapy.

Cognitive Therapy

"Cognitive therapy is a structured active short-term treatment for depression and anxiety which is based on helping the patient identify and change the distorted thought patterns that trigger and perpetuate his or her distress" (Childress and Burns 1981).

Rush et al. (1977) compared cognitive therapy to pharmacotherapy in the treatment of depression. Patients were randomly assigned to the two groups (19 and 22 respectively). Imipramine was the drug used. All patients showed a significant decrease in symptoms, but cognitive therapy provided the greater decrease by a wide margin. A reported 78.9% of cognitive therapy patients showed either "marked improvements" or complete symptom remission as compared with 22.7% of drug patients. Drop-out rates and numbers re-entering treatment also differed considerably. Rush et al. (1977) were enthusiastic about their results and considered cognitive therapy to be superior to all other types of treatment. Blackburn et al. (1981) noted that this formed a possible bias because the experiment was conducted at the centre for cognitive therapy and drugs may not have been prescribed with much conviction by non-blind therapists. Whereas the drugs used in the study of Blackburn et al. (1981) were "tailored" to each individual, imipramine was prescribed for all patients in the study of Rush et al. (1977). Beck himself is quoted by Bari Koalta (1981) as saying "Penn appears be to be mecca for cognitive therapy. Any study done here would be suspect unless it was replicated elsewhere."

Rush et al. reached similar conclusions in a study in 1982. The two concepts examined were hopelessness and self-concept. Cognitive therapy, which proposed to reduce negative views of self and future, was expected to be the more effective treatment in reducing these two symptoms, while imipramine was expected to help symptoms such as lack of sleep or appetite. Depressed outpatients, 18 in cognitive therapy and 17 on drugs, were treated for approximately 11 weeks with one or other of the treatments. Drug patients also saw a clinician once a week for 20 minutes for a loosely supportive session. The measures used were the hopelessness scale, the Miskimins Self Goal Other Part II and, to gauge improvement, the Hamilton Rating Scale for depression.

By attempting to correlate the results of the other scales with the Hamilton scale, it was found that the hopelessness scale was related to overall depressive symptoms, whereas the self-concept scale, which did not correlate, appeared to be of "a different dimension." Cognitive therapy again had better results than pharmacotherapy, with greater improvements for hopelessness and more generalized gain with self-concept. An important clinical implication for these findings is that hopelessness and suicidal intent have a high correlation. Therefore, if cognitive therapy can produce a greater reduction in hopelessness than imipramine can, it may consequently reduce suicidal intent as well.

The same group, in a paper by Kovacs et al. (1981), tested cognitive therapy and imipramine on 44 depressed patients. Again, cognitive therapy proved superior as regards symptomatic improvement and a considerably higher treatment completion rate. This result was found to be maintained at a 1-year follow-up.

Woody et al. (1983) found cognitive-behavioural therapy and drug counselling to be better than drug counselling alone in the treatment of drug addicts. However, it did not prove as effective as supportive-expressive therapy in this case.

Weissman's (1979) review cited six studies in the area of cognitive therapy, five of which were completed at that time. Two studies showed cognitive therapy to be the superior treatment and the remaining three showed cognitive therapy in combination with other types of therapy to be superior as well. The subjects were all depressed patients.

The evidence of the reviewed literature seems to indicate very strongly the efficacy of cognitive therapy, especially in the case of depression.

Blackburn et al. (1981) compared cognitive therapy to pharmacotherapy and looked at the two in combination. Sixty-four depressed patients were selected ultimately from either hospitals or general practice and all were rated on seven different measures of mood. Patients were then randomly divided into the three groups. The results proved cognitive therapy to be superior to the drug treatment in general practice only, but the combination treatment was superior to drugs alone for those in hospital and in general practice. General practice patients responded more quickly to treatment and were exposed to less situational stress factors than hospital patients.

Personal Construct Therapy

Bannister (1983) described a relatively new type of therapy which had been developed from Kelly's original theory of personal constructs. The problems patients display originate from the continual cyclical use of weak constructs they have built to cope with "reality." A troubled person is not consistent in his or her way of looking at the world and it is the aim of the personal construct therapist to help adjust the patient's world structures and to break the vicious circle of using invalid constructs. The interpretation a person places on situations, experiences, feelings or events are seen as most important here. By definition, the therapist is also using his constructs on "reality," and this fact must also be taken into account. Research with construct pschotherapy has been done in the areas of stuttering, depression, schizophrenic thought disorder, alcoholism, suicide and family therapy. Gwynne Jones (1978) reviewed construct therapy in a discussion on psychological treatment methods for schizophrenia. He was of the opinion that personal construct therapy is a promising area for the treatment of schizophrenia. Bannister tested his theories "by attempting to produce a specific area of ‚thought disorder' in normal subjects by ‚controlled validation' and ‚invalidation' of their judgements from photographs of people in terms of provided constructs. As predicted the relationships between serially invalidated constructs became progressively closer to random."

Bannister proceeded to test his feelings with schizophrenic patients by attempting to decrease their thought disorders. The results of a 2-year trial with a control group were inconclusive. However, Bannister felt this was due to lack of environmental control.

Family Therapy

Leff et al. (1982) explored social intervention with 24 families of schizophrenic patients, 12 families being assigned to routine outpatient care and 12 to social intervention. The selection criterion for families was high "expressed emotion" on the part of the relatives with whom they had a lot of contact. The social intervention took the form of an educational programme, a relatives' group and family sessions. The relatives' group was included so that relatives with high expressed emotions could see how relatives with low epressed emotions coped, and hopefully learn from them. All patients remained on medication.

The results showed social intervention to be a success; this finding provides evidence for the causal role in relapse of relatives' expressed emotion, as schizophrenic patients whose families received therapy relapsed significantly less than the control group.

Epstein and Vlok (1981) used a review by Gurman and Kniskern exclusively in their section on family therapy. Gurman and Kniskern looked at some 200 studies and their findings were extremely positive for family therapy. Every study which compared family therapy with other types of treatment showed it to be equal or superior. Although length of treatment was not shown to be a factor determining success, the presence of both spouses was. There are also indications of success with physical problems such as anorexia and drug abuse.

Goldstein et al. (1978) also looked at family therapy and use of drugs on 104 acute young schizophrenic patients in after care. No patients who had received high drug doses and family therapy relapsed, while 48% of those who received a low drug dose and no therapy did. The type of family therapy they found so effective was crisis orientated.

Lesser (1979) reviewed Compley's study of a non-random population of 42 families with a matched control group to examine family therapy as a technique for dealing with emotional problems in family medicine. "The results indicated that patients treated with family therapy placed 50% fewer demands on the physician and clinic than patients in the control groups treated with either medication, and/or psychotherapy by the family physician."

Cost Effectiveness and Cost Benefit Studies

There have been many attempts to prove the efficacy of psychotherapy, but another important question which has been asked after "will it work?", is "how much will it cost?" or "is it economical?" Studies of efficacy are often undertaken at the request of a government to see if state funding should be made available. The "mega trial" by the NIMH is an example of such an undertaking. Medical insurance companies also seek to determine cost as well as efficacy. Comparison trials are of particular importance here, and if one psychotherapy is proved to be more beneficial than another it may be chosen over others as the treatment for which reimbursement for example may be given. Ordinary clinical trials performed under laboratory conditions do not give indications of cost in day-to-day institutions.

Parloff (1980) commented that "demonstrating that psychotherapy reduces the misuse of medical facilities would indeed be a pertinent argument for justifying inclusion of psychological therapies in comprehensive insurance plans."

Culliton and Waterfall (1980) reviewed the reasons for the results of the NIMH's clinical trial which Parloff headed. The motivation for the study came from the American Federal Health Agency whose policies on health are often copied by the major insurance companies. Without convincing evidence of psychotherapy's worth it was suggested that these companies might neglect or even fail to cover mental health treatment at all. Although the results were not clear cut, and precise answers were not given as to what works and for whom, the overall worth of psychotherapy was felt to be proven. Psychotherapy was found better than spontaneous remission and some guidelines were given.

Follette and Cummings (1967) showed that people who avail themselves of psychiatric services also use other medical services to a significant degree, but it was not known whether "the provision of psychiatric services is associated with a reduction of medical services utilisation (defined as visits to other medical clinics, outpatient, laboratory and x-ray procedures, and days of hospitalisation)." At the time of the study (1959–1964) psychiatry was not covered on a prepaid basis by the health plan of the area (Northern California). One hundred and fifty patients were selected, of whom 80 had one interview only. 41 were seen for two to eight interviews (short-term) and 31 were seen for nine or more interviews (long-term). A control group was selected from medical records. "The results of the study indicated a significant decline in medical utilisation in the psychotherapy groups when compared to the control groups." The one visit and short-term groups utilized services less than the long-term group in the sense that long-term patients appeared to substitute psychiatric services for medical care. The findings remained constant for the 5 years of the study.

Cummings (1977) noted that due to the comparative ease of obtaining medical care, many people visit doctors for complaints which, although no less trivial are often a plea for help or understanding of an emotional disorder, i.e. psychosomatic. Cummings' point is that making psychotherapy available through health systems can only be economical as it is "more than offset by savings in medical utilistion." National Health insurers cannot favour one illness over another in this field. "The implications for National Health Insurance are that the inclusion of an appropriate realistic psychotherapy benefit is both essential and economically feasible."

Goldberg et al. (1970) also looked at the effect of psychiatric therapy on the utilization of medical services. The therapy was short term and the setting was a prepaid group practice medical programme, and 256 outpatients participated. Although a control group as such was not employed the records of the subjects' previous history of utilization sufficed. These patients showed a marked reduction in their utilization of physician services, laboratory and X-ray procedures compared with the year before the study. In terms of visits made the reduction was approximately 30% for each service.

Lesser (1979) was concerned with psychotherapy benefits in Canada and reviewed, among other aspects, cost benefit studies. Lesser began by quoting from a report by the group on the advancement of psychiatry and noted that "the utilisation cost benefit argument is that for certain groups of patients this treatment (psychotherapy) is less costly than any available alternative."

Lesser reviewed the studies by Follette and Cummings (1967) and Goldberg et al. (1970) and noted several drawbacks in them, such as screening, inadequate representation of all social classes, inadequate or absent control groups and the possibility that patients could have received help other than that given in the study. Studies such as those of Comley, Jameson, Shuman and Young, Duherssen et al. (West Germany) and Sharfstein were cited for the recommendations for future research.

Lesser's main conclusion was that "psychotherapy cost benefit studies provide compelling evidence that brief psychotherapy definitely reduces medical costs. The situation is less clear regarding intensive long term therapy where the costs of hospitalisation only are significantly reduced." He also strongly recomended the practice of peer review, especially for long-term cases.

Bordaty and Andrews (1983) compared patients receiving brief problem-orientated dynamic psychotherapy with patients receiving family practitioner therapy and with patients receiving no therapy. All patients came from suburban family practices. All patients improved, but no group improved more than another. However, the authors recommended that primary care physicians should develop effective techniques as the family practitioner is the first person patients turn to and the specialist mental health services of Australia would be unable to cope with the estimated 15% of the population who would need psychological help in the next year.

As one estimate suggests, 60% of medical visits are for somatic complaints so greater utilization of psychotherapeutic services must be advantageous. Establishing psychotherapy in medical programmes and insurance schemes should improve the authority and reliability of psychotherapy. Psychotherapy would then be available and more accessible to a wider proportion of the population.

Other Factors

Predictions of Success

Various attempts have been made to predict the outcome of psychotherapy and to discover which factors involved in the process make the best predicters.

Blau (1950) derived a formula for success prediction from previous clients' statements and tested it with "the resulting co- efficient correlation of 0.90 between prediction formula values and ratings of therapy success." Although the correlation was significant the sample was extremely limited and therefore prediction value can only be seen as an indicator. Further research was planned.

Fiske et al. (1964) attempted to predict change in psychotherapy using composite raw and residual scores. Based on factor analysis there were 21 correlations between criteria, and 17 of these gave positive although low results. No criterion was found to be a better predictor than another, and no one criterion was sufficient alone. The authors did not consider the experiment a success and suggested an entirely different approach to the problem.

Greenspan and Sharfstein (1981) put forward the idea that each psychotherapeutic approach should outline "process steps," and stated that "the capacity to predict a relationship between process and outcome at each stage in a therapeutic procedure is the relevant test of efficacy."

Predictions from the Penn psychotherapy project by Luborsky et al. (1980) were drawn from two sources, direct predictions by patients, therapists and clinical observers, and predictive measures derived from the same sources. The success of the latter was generally insignificant while clinical observers' predictions were highest. The therapist and patient ratings were not significant. They concluded that "the final outcomes of psychotherapy appear to be predictable from some types of initial information but only at very insignificant levels."

So many factors appear to be involved in the outcome of psychotherapy that prediction of success has been found to be a virtually impossible task. It would appear that ratings made by therapists themselves are not reliable. The ability to predict success surely involves an understanding of all the factors involved in a therapeutic relationship and the power to manipulate these.

Psychotherapist Variable

The two most important factors in a psychotherapeutic relationship are, naturally, the patient and the therapist. Intelligent, highly motivated patients are the "best" patients, but what makes a good therapist, which college he or she went to, which therapy he or she uses, or simply how good a listener he or she is? The literature more often focuses on which therapy is the best, but a few studies do take account of the factors involved in a therapeutic relationship.

Borus et al. (1979) looked at the role of the therapist and examined whether being an indigenous therapist was an advantage or a disadvantage. On the one hand, an indigenous therapist has valuable background knowledge into the particular social problems of the area. In simple terms, he speaks the same language as his patients and has "longitudinal knowledge." On the other hand, role blurring causes the loss of a lot of clinical objectivity. The therapists found that they could not successfully treat friends or neighbours. Patients commented that they did not trust the therapist to be completely confidential about their problems in an area where everyone knows everyone else. They knew the life history of the therapist and could not feel the same respect as they would for an outsider. The professionalism of the relationship between therapist and patient was lost and it would seem that therapy cannot be effective without it.

Borus et al. (1979) rejected the usefulness of indigeneity to a therapist and listed important characteristics as sensitivity to other's problems, the ability to show empathy, and the ability to translate psychosocial concepts to patients etc.

Chevron and Rounsaville (1983) evaluated the clinical skills of nine psychotherapists using didactic examination, global ratings, supervisor's ratings, therapists' self-ratings and independent evaluators' ratings of video-taped sessions. The results showed a very poor level of agreement among the five ratings. The only ratings to correlate with patient outcome were the supervisors'.

Weissman et al. (1982) described the issues involved in training experienced psychotherapists to participate in outcome studies. Conflict areas between research and clinical goals, and therapists' expectations are research restrictions, the restriction to a defined psychotherapy, and therapists' feelings about being evaluated.

Luborsky et al. (1971) reviewed 166 studies and under the heading of therapist variables found the positive factors to be experience, attitude and interest patterns, empathy and similarity of patient and therapist.

Strupp and Hadley (1979) found that patients treated by college professors improved just as well as those treated by professional psychotherapists. However, the patients were only mildly neurotic and the therapy was of short duration.

Emanuel (1983) gave much more emphasis to the therapist than the therapy. He saw psychotherapy as an art or skill that cannot be taught but rather is innate.

Parloff (1976) concluded his comprehensive review of psychotherapies with the comment, "psychotherapy is mediated by the individual and further modified by the nature of the interaction with the particular patient."

Evaluation of Psychotherapy

Varying methods have been employed in the numerous attempts that have been made of the evaluation of psychotherapy. Some of these are outlined below.

Bloch et al. (1977) attempted to measure outcome by means of independent judges. Twenty-seven neurotic patients and 42 psychotherapists took part. The latter were split into teams of three and viewed videotapes of therapy sessions without receiving any information about them. Lists of problems were drawn up individually and later pooled for each team. However, agreement about both clinical states and their outcome was found to be poor. Two of the factors accounting for this were that large differences were found in terminology and the fact that some psychotherapists clustered several problems into one. The authors commented that the general lack of agreement of a standard of reliability posed a great problem for researchers as, however rigorous they themselves may consider their own measures to be, other parties invariably find some objection which casts doubt on the findings.

Kazdin and Wilson (1978) claimed that multiple criteria are needed to evaluate treatments. They criticized the use of the average patient performance measure so often employed in clinical trials. They pointed to no less than 11 criteria which they considered essential for a thorough evaluation. The first three were amount of patient change (across groups), alternate measures of outcome, and measures related to efficiency, cost and patient evaluation of treatment. Patient-related criteria were clinical importance of therapeutic change, proportion of patients who improve, breadth and durability of the improvements and acceptability of the treatment to patients. Criteria concerned with evaluations of different therapies were duration of different treatments, efficacy and costs of administration of treatment, financial and emotional cost to the patient, and cost as related to overall effectiveness.

London and Klerman (1982) outlined a need for a body for psychotherapy similar to the Food and Drug Administration Board in the United States.

They did not see psychotherapy as restrictable to the health professions and believed that the boundary between research and practice was as clear for psychotherapy as for any health intervention. The criteria involved in delineating this boundary were intent, authority and "routine and accepted practice." Outcome was seen only as a desired rather than an existing criterion. Establishing psychotherapy's efficacy was seen as a most pressing problem.

Factors in Psychotherapy

Strupp and Hadley (1979) compared specific and nonspecific factors in psychotherapy by comparing the outcome of patients treated either by college professors or by experienced psychotherapists. No differences in success were found between the two groups and they concluded that "positive changes are generally attributable to the healing effects of a benign human relationship." Success, therefore, involved a highly motivated patient who took advantage of a therapeutic relationship in which he or she perceived the therapist's intervention as an expression of caring and genuine interest.

Frank (1971) commented that dominant trends in psychotherapy appear to follow those of cultural attitudes and values. Often the same techniques are being employed but under new names. He matched four factors determining psychological distress to four treatments: first, constitutional vulnerabilities to be treated by drugs; secondly, environmental crises requiring simple emotional support; thirdly existential anxieties needing spiritual guidance; and fourthly, warping of early life experiences, this being the only one requiring trained psychotherapists to correct "faulty learned perceptual and behavioural habits."

Garfield (1973) criticized Strupp's article (1973) "on the basic ingredients of psychotherapy" for overemphasizing the importance of a client in such a way as to make only intelligent motivated patients worthy of psychotherapy. While conceding that the patient variable is a very important one, he felt Strupp's presentation of the case was limiting and restrictive of psychotherapy.

Practitioners' Views

Chodoff (1982) believed large-scale trials to be of little relevance to practising outpatient clinics. The experience of practitioners, however, he felt to be of some value. He saw psychotherapy as effective with emotional crises, in improving the life-quality of physically handicapped people, with problems of ageing and with schizophrenia. He had seen much success of psychotherapy with symptomatic neuroses or sexual dysfunctions. He claimed that predictability of psychotherapy is equally poor in practice as it is in research experiments.

Parloff (1984) agreed with Chodoff that research and practice were too separate and the problem as he saw it was that therapists' practices were difficult to study in a controlled manner and the findings of the researchers were too distantly related to everyday business to be of any use. Therapists saw psychotherapy as an art whereas researchers saw it as a science or a quasi-science.

Emanuel (1983) also doubted the value of clinical trials because of the "fluidity of psychiatric diagnosis" and the difficulty of isolating the variables in "therapeutic confrontations." For Emanuel, psychotherapy is an art and a talent which cannot be either taught or learnt. Listening to patients is most important to Emanuel, who prefers to guide rather than to direct them.

Outcome

Although many of the articles reviewed so far involve outcome in psychotherapy, the papers in this section relate more specifically to this area.

Adams (1978) disagreed with Bloch et al. (1977) in directing attention to assessing improvement after treatment. Adams felt it was the severity of patients' problems which should be assessed. One reason was that severity of a problem is often the criterion for admissions and discharges. The reliability of severity as an outcome measure should be greater.

Cristol (1972) reviewed 15 selected studies of outcome. He found that even though proper psychological tests were employed change was not demonstrated. He also found that the studies did not prove either insight or behaviour therapy (alone or in combination) to be more effective than the spontaneous remission rate.

Luborsky et al. (1971) reviewed 166 studies concerned with prediction outcome of individual psychotherapy. The influential factors were thought to be in the areas of the patient, therapist and treatment. Most studies involved patient factors and the variables associated with positive change were adequacy of personality functioning, absence of schizoid tendencies, motivation, intelligence, anxiety, and educational and social assets. Positive therapist variables were experience, attitude and interest patterns, empathy and patient-therapist similarity. The only positive treatment variable was the number of sessions involved.

Drug Abuse

Two papers dealing with the subject of drug abuse are reviewed here. The first of these is by Luborsky and McLellan (1978), who were concerned with predicting the outcome of psychological treatments. They reported their own study of 50 opiate addicts and reviewed several others. They concluded that they were unable to predict the outcome of psychotherapy and the patients themselves appeared to be more accurate in this area.

Woody et al. (1983) divided 110 subjects into three groups, those receiving (1) cognitive-behavioural therapy plus counselling (39), (2) supportive and expressive counselling (32), and (3) drug counselling (39). All patients were maintained on methadone throughout the 6-month study. Precautions were successfully undertaken to ensure that patients kept appointments and that the therapists' morale did not suffer. All patients improved to some extent on many of the outcome measures, though patients receiving psychotherapy and counselling made more and larger gains than patients with drug counselling alone. Of the two psychotherapies the supportive, expressive group was found to be superior. On the drug-use factor patients receiving supportive, expressive and drug counselling improved more than did those who had the cognitive-behavioural therapy. The authors attributed the superiority of the psychotherapists to the fact that the therapists were able "to form a relationship combined with special knowledge and skill about how to use it," whereas counsellors had trouble managing some patients, especially very disturbed cases. The results held throughout the 7-month follow-up.

Client-Centred Therapy

Rogers (1957) asked "Is it possible to state, in terms which are clearly definable and measurable, the psychological conditions which are both necessary and sufficient to bring about constructive personality change?". In answering this question he listed six such conditions:

1. The two persons are in psychological contact
2. The "client" is in a state of incongruence
3. The "therapist" is congruent or integrated in the relationship
4. The therapist experiences unconditional positive regard for the client
5. The therapist experiences an empathic understanding of the client's internal frame of reference and endeavours to communicate this experience to the client
6. Communication to the client of the therapist's empathic understanding and unconditional positive regard is, to a minimal degree, achieved.

Rogers stated that "no other conditions are necessary ... the process of constructive personality change will follow."

Relaxation Therapy

Brauer et al. (1979) used three conditions in their experiment to test relaxation therapy for hypertension. These were relaxation training with the therapist, relaxation training by means of audio cassette, and non-specific individual therapy. No immediate differences were found between the three groups, but after 6 months the first group (relaxation training with the therapist) displayed a significant decrease in diastolic blood pressure. The results proved that the relaxation therapy's efficacy was due to the training procedures and not to non-specific factors.

Telephone Prompting

Burgoyne et al. (1983) conducted an investigation with the hypothesis that telephone prompting increased attendance at the first appointment at the clinics. Their finding was, however, that social economic factors such as having a telephone were related to increased attendance rather than telephone prompting alone. Therefore, ascertaining whether a patient owned a telephone identified patients who were likely to keep their first appointment. They advised caution in interpreting results in this area.

Access to Records

Roth et al. (1980) reviewed their personal experiences of allowing or not allowing patients access to their own records. In general, the practice was considered beneficial and certainly not harmful in almost all cases. The presence of the therapist or one who understood the record was considered essential for purposes of explanation and support. Legal and moral questions arose if information from other people about the patients was present in the record.

Attitudinal Changes

Kane et al. (1983) undertook a study to assess attitudinal changes in involuntarily committed patients after treatment. A relationship between change of attitude and patient characteristics or treatment outcome was sought. It was found that those patients achieving symptom remissions were most likely to have positive attitudes and that older patients changed attitudes less quickly. Schizophrenic patients showed no significant difference in any area from other patients, except that they were more optimistic about the benefits of being committed.

McCord (1978) reported the findings of the follow-up of an extremely complex 5-year trial, the Cambridge Summerville Youth Study. Several hundreds of both "difficult" and "average" boys were recommended to the programme, where they and their families received either some kind of therapeutic intervention or no intervention. Thirty years later, approximately half of the participants were traced and followed up. Subjective evaluation by the treated group was the only measurement to indicate any positive effects of intervention, however, and there were some negative side-effects such as increased criminal behaviour, lowered occupational status and decreased job satisfaction. McCord felt the social programme should be reviewed although not necessarily ceased. It should be noted that the type of intervention used in the study was never specified.

Conclusion

In a recent review of psychotherapy research and its incredible credibility crises, Parloff challenged the glib interpretation of the research evidence as demonstrating that "all psychotherapies work and all work equally well." His reservations were based largely on the fact that the literature suggesting this does not adequately represent the non-behavioural therapies, typical patients, or fully trained therapists. Furthermore, outcome measures did not attempt to assess "internal" change claimed by the psychodynamic therapies. He felt that much more research was required into the efficacy of psychodynamically orientated psychotherapy. Too often in the past studies have been methodologically correct but not meaningful in that the measures used have been insufficiently comprehensive.

A particular problem in psychodynamic psychotherapy is that the aims are often broad ranging. Outcome measures must be devised to reflect this since the narrow symptom scores appropriate in pharmacological studies cannot purport to do so. An epidemiological approach may be more useful, using objective measures such as utilization of medical services or recidivism in the case of self-poisoning.

The multicentre trial is a technique that could be much more widely used, and may be suitable for international action. The evaluation of the skill of the psychotherapist also requires much further work in the light of allegations of negative effects.

Above all, psychotherapy research for the future will require interdisciplinary collaboration, more generous support of studies provided that their methodology is rigorous, and, hopefully, international co-operation.

References

Adams M (1978) How should we measure outcome in psychotherapy? Br J Psychiatry 132:595–597

Ayllon T, Azrin NH (1968) The token economy: a motivational system for therapy and rehabilitation. Appleton-Century-Crofts, New York

Andrews G, Harvey R (1981) Does psychotherapy benefit neurotic patients? Arch Gen Psychiatry 38:1203–1208

Baehr G (1954) The comparative effectiveness of individual psychotherapy, group psychotherapy, and a combination of these methods. J Consult Psychol 18:179–183

Bannister D (1983) Personal construct psychotherapy. Br J Hosp Med 30:72–74

Bari Koalta G (1981) Clinical trial of psychotherapies is under way. Science 212:432–433

Beck J, Golden S, Arnold F (1981) An empirical investigation of psychotherapy with schizophrenic patients. Schizophr Bull 7:241–247

Blackburn I, Bishop S, Glen A, Whalley L, Christie J (1981) The efficacy of cognitive therapy in depression: a treatment trial using cognitive therapy and pharmacotherapy, each alone and in combination. Br J Psychiatry 139:181–189

Blau T (1950) Report on a method of predicting success in psychotherapy. J Clin Psychol 6:403–406

Bloch S, Bond F, Qualls B, Yalam I, Zimmerman E (1977) Outcome in psychotherapy evaluated by independent judges. Br J Psychiatry 131:410–414

Borus J, Anastasia M, Casoni R, Dello Russo R, DiMascio L, Fusco L, Rubenstein J, Snyder M (1979) Psychotherapy in the goldfish bowl.Arch Gen Psychiatry 36:187–190

Bovill D (1977) An outcome study of group psychotherapy. Br J Psychiatry 131:95–98

Brauer A, Horlick L, Nelson E, Farquhar J, Agras W (1979) Relaxation therapy for essential hypertension: a veterans administration outpatient study. J Behav Med 2:21–29

Bordaty H, Andrews G (1983) Brief psychotherapy in family practice. Br J Psychiatry 143:11–19

Burgoyne R, Acosta F, Yamatomo J (1983) Telephone prompting to increase attendance at a psychiatric outpatient clinic. Am J Psychiatry 140:345–347

Burke J, White H, Havens L (1979) Which shortterm therapy? Arch Gen Psychiatry 36:177–186
Chevron E, Rounsaville B (1983) Evaluating the clinical skills of psychotherapists: a comparison of techniques. Arch Gen Psychiatry 40:1129–1132
Childress A, Burns D (1981) The basics of cognitive therapy. Psychosomatics 22:1017–1027
Chodoff P (1982) Assessment of psychotherapy: reflections of a practitioner. Arch Gen Psychiatry 39:1097–1103
Cristol A (1972) Studies of outcome of psychotherapy. Compr Psychiatry 13:189–200
Culliton B, Waterfall W (1980) Assessing the benefits. Br Med J 280:917–918
Cummings N (1977) The anatomy of psychotherapy under National Health Insurance. Am Psychol 32:711–718
Dagadakis C, Hunt D, Carr J (1981) Pragmatic issues in design and implementation of a psychotherapy outcome study. Hosp Commun Psychiatry 32:858–861
Daly R (1983) Special problems in evaluation of psychotherapy. In: Helgason T (ed) Methodology in evaluation of psychiatric treatment. Cambridge University Press, pp 123–136
Daly R (1984) Psychotherapy of schizophrenia. In: Helgason T (ed) Needed areas of research on long-term treatment of functional psychoses. Cambridge University Press, pp 59–76
Earll L, Kincey J (1982) Clinical psychology in general practice: a controlled trial evaluation. J R Coll Gen Pract 32:32–37
Ellis A (1957) Outcome of employing three techniques of psychotherapy. J Clin Psychol 13:344–350
Emanuel E (1983) Some thoughts about psychotherapy. Can Med Ass J 128:460–464
Epstein N, Vlok L (1981) Research on the results of psychotherapy. Am J Psychiatry 138:1027–1035
Eysenck H (1952) The effects of psychotherapy: an evaluation. J Consult Clin Psychol 16:319–324
Eysenck H (1965) The effects of psychotherapy. Int J Psychiatry 1:99–142
Fiske D, Cartwright D, Kirtner W (1964) Are psychotherapeutic changes predictable? J Abnor Soc Psychol 69:418–426
Follette W, Cummings N (1967) Psychiatric services and medical utilization in a prepaid health plan setting. Med Care 5:25–35
Frank J (1971) Therapeutic factors in psychotherapy. Am J Psychother 25:350–361
Garfield S (1973) Basic ingredients of common factors in psychotherapy? J Consult Clin Psychol 41:9–12
Gelder M, Marks I, Wolff H, Clarke M (1967) Desensitization and psychotherapy in the treatment of phobic states: a controlled inquiry. Br J Psychiatry 113:53–73
Gillan P, Rachman S (1974) An experimental investigation of desensitization in phobic patients. Br J Psychiatry 124:392–401
Glass R (1984) Psychotherapy – scientific art or artistic science? Arch Gen Psychiatry 41:525–526
Goldberg I, Krantz G, Locke B (1970) Effect of a short-term out-patient psychiatric therapy benefit on the utilization of medical services in a prepaid group practice medical program. Med Care 8:419–428
Goldfried M (1982) On the history of therapeutic integration. Behav Ther 13:572–593
Greenspan S, Sharfstein S (1981) efficacy of psychotherapy: a: asking the right questions. Arch Gen Psychiatry 38:1213–1219
Gwynne-Jones H (1978) Psychological aspects of treatment of in-patients. In: Wing J (ed) Schizophrenia: towards a new synthesis. Academic Press, pp 189–209
Hogarty GE, Goldberg SC (1973) Drugs and sociotherapy in the post hospital maintenance of schizophrenic patients: 1 year relapse rates. Arch Gen Pschiatr 28:54
Hussain M (1971) Desensitization and flooding (implosion) in treatment of phobias. Am J Psychiatry 127:1509–1514
Kane J, Quitkin F, Rifkin A, Wegner J, Roenberg G, Borenstein M (1983). Attitudinal changes of involuntarily committed patients following treatment. Arch Gen Psychiatry 40:374–377

Kazdin A, Wilson G (1978) Criteria for evaluating psychotherapy. Arch Gen Psychiatry 35:407–416
Kelly GA (1955) The psychology of personal constructs, vols 1 and 2. Northon, London New York
Klein D, Zitrin C, Waerner M, Ross D (1983) Treatment of phobias: 2. Arch Gen Psychiatry 40:139–145
Klerman G, DiMascio A, Weissman M, Prusoff B, Paykel E (1974) Treatment of depression by drugs and psychotherapy. Am J Psychiatry 131:186–191
Kovacs M, Rush A, Beck A, Hollon S (1981) Depressed outpatients treated with cognitive therapy or pharmacotherapy: a one-year follow-up. Arch Gen Psychiatry 38:33–39
Lazarus A (1963) The results of behaviour therapy in 126 cases of severe neurosis. Behav Res Ther 1:69–79
Leff J, Kuipers L, Berkowitz R, Eberlein-Vries R, Sturgeon D (1982) A controlled trial of social intervention in the families of schizophrenic patients. Br J Psychiatry 141:121–134
Lesser A (1979) Psychotherapy, benefits and costs. Psychiatr J Univ Ottawa 4:191–196
Lolas F, Mergenthaler E, Von Rad M (1982) Content analysis of verbal behaviour in psychotherapy research: a comparison between two methods. Br J Med Psychol 55:327–333
London P, Klerman G (1982) Evaluating psychotherapy. Am J Psychiatry 139:709–717
Luborsky L, McLellan A (1978) Our suprising in ability to predict the outcomes of psychological treatments. Am J Drug Alcohol Abuse 5:387–398
Luborsky L, Chandler M, Auerbach A, Cohen J, Bachrach H (1971) Factors influencing the outcome of psychotherapy. Psychol Bull 75:145–185
Luborsky L, Singer B, Luborsky L (1975) Comparative studies of psychotherapies – Is it true that "Everyone has won and all must have prizes?" Arch Gen Psychiatry 32:995–1002
Luborsky L, Mintz J, Auerbach A, Christoph C, Bachrach H, Todd T, Johnson M, Cohen M, O'Brien C (1980) Predicting the outcome of psychotherapy – Findings on the Penn psychotherapy project. Arch Gen Psychiatry 37:471–481
Malan D (1973) The outcome in psychotherapy research: a historical review. Arch Gen Psychiatry 29:719–729
Malan DH (1976) The frontier of brief psychotherapy. Plenum Medical Books, New York
Marks I (1976) The current status of behavioural psychotherapy: theory and practice. Am J Psychiatry 133:253–261
Marmor J (1971) Dynamic psychotherapy and behaviour therapy. Arch Gen Psychiatry 24:22–28
Marshall E (1980) Psychotherapy Works, but for whom? Science 207:506–508
Marziali E (1984) Prediction of outcome of brief psychotherapy from therapist interpretive interventions. Arch Gen Psychiatry 41:301–304
May P (1973) Research in psychotherapy and psychoanalysis. Int J Psychiatry 11:78–86
May P (1980) Schizophrenia: evaluation of treatment methods. In: Kaplan, Freedman, Sadock (eds) Comprehensive textbook of psychiatry vol III. Williams and Wilkins, Baltimore pp 2151–2175
McCord J (1978) A thirty-year follow-up of treatment effects. Am Psychol 33:284–289
McGlashan T (1982) DSM-111 schizophrenia and individual psychotherapy. J Nerv Ment Dis 170:752–757
Mintz J, Luborsky L, Christoph P (1979) Measuring the outcomes of psychotherapy: findings of the Penn Psychotherapy project. J Consult Clin Psychol 47:319–334
O'Brien C, Hamm K, Ray B, Pierce J, Luborsky L, Mintz J (1972) Group vs individual psychotherapy with schizophrenics. Arch Gen Psychiatry 27:474–478
Parloff M (1976) Shopping for the right therapy. Saturday Rev 3:14–20
Parloff M (1980) Psychotherapy and research: an anaclitic depression. Psychiatry 43:279–292
Parloff MB (1984) Psychotherapy Research and its Incredible Credibility Crisis. Clin Psychol Rev 4:1–21

Prioleau L, Murdock M, Brody N (1983). An analysis of psychotherapy versus placebo studies. Behav Brain Sci 6:295–310

Rogers C (1957) The necessary and sufficient conditions of therapeutic personality change. J Consult Psychol 21:95–103

Roth L, Wolford J, Meisel A (1980) Patient access to records: tonic or toxin? Am J Psychiatry 137:592–596

Rounsaville B, Klerman G, Weissman M (1981) Do psychotherapy and pharmacotherapy for depression conflict? empirical evidence from a clinical trial. Arch Gen Psychiatry 38:24–29

Rush A, Beck A, Kovacs M, Hollon S (1977) Comparative efficacy of cognitive therapy and pharmacotherapy in the treatment of depressed outpatients. Cognitive Ther Res 1:17–37

Rush A, Beck A, Kovacs M, Weissenburger J, Hollon S (1982) Comparison of the effects of cognitive therapy and pharmacotherapy on hopelessness and self-concept. Am J Psychiatry 139:862–866

Segraves R, Smith R (1976) Concurrent psychotherapy and behaviour therapy. Arch Gen Psychiatry 33:756–763

Shepherd M (1984) What price psychotherapy? Br Med J 288:309–310

Sifneos PE (1973) Short term psychotherapy and emotional crisis. Harvard University Press, Cambridge

Sloane R, Staples F, Cristol A, Yorkston N, Whipple K (1975) Short-term analytically oriented psychotherapy versus behaviour therapy. Am J Psychiatry 132:373–377

Smith ML (1982) What research says about the effectiveness of psychotherapy. Hosp Commun Psychiatry 33:457–461

Smith ML, Glass GV (1977) Meta-analysis of psychotherapy outcome studies. Am Psychol 32:752–760

Smith ML, Glass GV, Miller TI (1980) The benefits of psychotherapy. Johns Hopkins University Press, Baltimore

Strupp H (1973) The interpersonal relationship as a vehicle for therapeutic learning. J Consult Clin Psychol 41:13–15

Strupp H (1980a) Success and failure in time-limited psychotherapy: a systematic comparison of two gases: comparison 1. Arch Gen Psychiatry 37:595–603

Strupp H (1980b) Success and failure in time-limited psychotherapy: a systematic comparison of two cases: comparison 2. Arch Gen Psychiatry 37:708–716

Strupp H (1980c) Success and failure in time-limited psychotherapy: with special reference to the performance of a lay counselor (3). Arch Gen Psychiatry 37:831–841

Strupp H (1980a) Success and failure in time-limited psychotherapy: further evidence – comparison 4. Arch Gen Psychiatry 37:947–954

Strupp H, Hadley S (1979) Specific vs nonspecific factors in psychotherapy. Arch Gen Psychiatry 36:1125–1136

Vaughn CE, Leff JP (1976) The influence of family and source factors on the course of psychiatric illness: a comparison of schizophrenia and depressed neurotic patients. Br J Psychiatr 129:125–137

Weissman M (1979) The psychological treatment of depression: evidence for the efficacy of psychotherapy alone, in comparison with, and in combination with pharmacotherapy. Arch Gen Psychiatry 36:1261–1269

Weissman M, Rounsaville B, Chevron E (1982) Training psychotherapists to participate in psychotherapy outcome studies. Am J Psychiatry 139:1442–1446

Woody G, Luborsky L, McLellan A, O'Brien C, Beck A, Blaine J, Herman I, Hole A (1983) Psychotherapy for opiate addicts: does it help? Arch Gen Psychiatry 40:639–645

Research Strategies and Design in Psychological Treatments for Mental Illness: Review of the Nordic Literature

J.-O. OTTOSSON[1]

Introduction

This review will focus on the psychological treatment of schizophrenic disorders. In addition, studies from my own institution on the psychological treatment of phobic and psychosomatic disorders are summarized but not critically reviewed as are outcome studies on drug abuse.

Phobic Disorders

Four types of treatment which were given for 3 months with a 9-month follow-up period were compared. All patients received basal therapy in the form of standardized information, self-exposure instructions and anxiolytic medication. On group received this treatment only at monthly appointments (B). The others also received either therapist-directed prolonged exposure in vivo (PE), dynamically oriented supportive therapy (ST) or relaxation therapy (R). The outcome was assessed with a rating scale for phobic disordes (Alström et al. 1983).

In agoraphobic women rated unsuitable for insight-oriented psychotherapy (Persson and Alström 1983) all groups were about equally improved at the termination of treatment, with some advantage for PE and ST. At follow-up the ST group, had improved more than the other groups, the R group had improved least and the PE group shown some deterioration. ST, which took into account the overall adjustment as well as the symptoms, was thus the most successful treatment but this superiority did not manifest itself until the end of the follow-up period (Alström et al. 1984a).

In social phobic men and women rated unsuitable for insight-oriented psychotherapy, the phobia variables were more improved in the PE and ST groups than in the R and B groups at the termination of treatment. Although some deterioration occurred in the PE group during follow-up, the improvement in the target phobia was better than in the other groups. There were almost no improvements in the R and B groups. The ST and PE groups also showed improved social function while the global rating showed most im-

[1] Dept. of Psychiatry, Sahlgren Hospital, University of Gothenburg, S-41345 Gothenburg

Psychological Treatment of Mental Illness
Edited by R. J. Daly and E. A. Sand

provement in the PE group. In contrast to agoraphobic syndromes where ST turned out to be the best treatment, PE is superior in social phobic states. This may be because circumscribed phobias are generally best treated with behaviour therapies and the social phobias studied here were more circumscribed than the agoraphobias (Alström et al. 1984b).

Agoraphobic women rated suitable for insight-oriented psychotherapy who received non-insight-oriented types of treatment (PE, B and R) none the less showed clinically relevant improvement. This indicates a favourable prognosis for patients suitable for insight-oriented psychotherapy irrespective of mode of treatment. However, since the PE group was least improved in some neurotic symptoms and displayed treatment drop-out and symptom substitution, this mode of treatment cannot be recommended for insight-suitable patients. R patients came out favourably, in contrast to the poor outcome with this therapy in patients not suitable for insight-oriented psychotherapy (Alström et al. 1984c).

The different response patterns in agoraphobic and social phobic syndromes indicate basically different features. This is further indicated by differences in family history, personal history, personality and the course of the disorder (Persson and Nordlund 1985).

Suitability for insight-oriented psychotherapy as a prognostic factor was further elucidated when pairs of phobic female patients suitable and not suitable for insight-oriented psychotherapy were formed with age, type of phobia, global rating of severity, therapist and type of therapy as matching variables. Patients suitable for insight-oriented psychotherapy improved more than patients who were not suitable. Since the greater improvement pertained to the target phobia, it is possible that the patients suitable for insight psychotherapy practised self-exposure to a greater degree than patients who were not suitable. If this is so, the results cannot be generalized to types of neurosis in which the solution of intrapsychic conflicts may be of central importance to improvement (Persson and Alström 1984a).

The pretreatment expectations of improvement were associated with outcome with unspecific therapies (B and R), while the effects of specific therapies overruled the effects of expectations. The outcome of the treatment was better if the character of the treatment was in line with expectations (Persson and Nordlund 1983; Persson and Alström 1984b). There were several other interactions between prognostic factors and type of treatment which should be taken into account in the choice and design of treatment (Persson 1984; Persson et al. 1984).

Psychosomatic Disorders

Two types of treatment given for 3 months with a 12-month follow-up period were compared in patients with peptic ulcer disease and irritable bowel syndrome. All patients received conventional medical treatment, and one group also received short-therm psychotherapy administered in 1-h weekly sessions. Assessments were made by independent raters and self-ratings.

Patients with peptic ulcer disease improved to a similar extent during treatment, but at follow-up there was a significant difference in favour of the psychotherapy group in several respects. Globally rated, 42% had improved in the psychotherapy group versus 28% in the control group. Confounding factors such as use of drugs, smoking and drinking habits, treatment outside the programme and exposure to life events could not account for the different outcome (Svendlund 1983).

In patients with irritable bowel syndrome there was a significant difference in favour of the psychotherapy group immediately after the treatment. The difference was more pronounced at follow-up, as the psychotherapy group showed further improvement while the control group showed some deterioration. Globally rated, 49% had improved in the psychotherapy group versus 10% in the control group. Again, confounding factors could not account for the different outcomes (Sjödin 1983).

In both psychosomatic disorders, increased self-confidence and coping ability seem to be relevant therapeutic mechanisms of action. In most cases the psychotherapy had to develop through phases of symptom orientation and support before conflicts could be focused. The character of this type of psychotherapy is compatible with its being administered by general practitioners and other non-specialists in psychiatry, provided that training and supervision by psychiatrists educated in psychotherapy can be arranged.

Drug Abuse

Treatment programmes that concentrate on ward structure and run on operant principles have shown that it is possible to motivate addicts to engage in activities other than and incompatible with drug-taking behaviour, as long as they are in the treatment programme (Götestam and Melin 1980). The relevance of such institutional programmes to adjustment to society remains to be shown. Besides, individual programmes have to be elaborated which take into account the development of coping behaviours which are positively reinforced in the patient's natural environment. On the basis of existing data it is not possible to recommend a behavioural approach to the treatment of drug abuse. However, the rapid growth of empirical knowledge in this field allows cautions optimism.

A different approach to the treatment of young drug abusers was assessed in a quasi-experimental study. Supportive and limit-setting milieu therapy combined with systematic individual and family therapy came out best in a psychedelic drug-using group, whereas opiate and central stimulant abusers had the best results in an intensive, confrontative therapeutic community using special intake procedures, spontaneous marathon-like groups and systematic individual and family therapy (Vaglum and Fossheim 1980).

Schizophrenic Disorders

In this section, data from three projects will be discussed according to theory, treatment, patients, controls (if any), outcome, authors' conclusions and my own comments. The authors whose work is discussed have kindly sent me their published and unpublished data and permitted me to report them. A fourth study with an intra-subject design has shown that the application of a token economy programme for chronic schizophrenic patients significantly increased the frequency of reinforced behaviours such as bed-making, unsolicited ingestion of medicine and washing of clothes (Öst et al. 1976).

Gaustad Project (Uglestad 1978)

Theory. Psychoanalytically oriented ego-supportive relation therapy. Four dimensions of the ego were paid attention to:
1. Autonomy in relation to the family
2. Competence in social function
3. Identity with regard to self-appreciation and reasonable realization of the self
4. Balance between control and outlet of drives of the id

Treatment. Individual psychotherapy, two sessions per week for at least 1 year.

Index Patients. Six male schizophrenic patients, aged 26–35 years, previous in-patient care 4.4–11.2 years.

Controls. Control group I: Six male schizophrenic patients, aged 26–39 years, previous in-patient care 3.1–9.8 years, matched pair-wise to the index patients. They received intensive milieu treatment, four group sessions per week for 1 year and family and social rehabilitation. Control group II: Twelve male schizophrenic patients in the course of rehabilitation. Discharge was planned in the near future.

Results. The number of patients who could be discharged after 2 and 4 years may be seen in Table 1.

Author's Conclusions. Psychological mindedness is necessary in the treatment of schizophrenia. A high proportion of young chronic psychotic patients are

Table 1. Outcome study (Uglestad 1978)

Type of psychotherapy	*N*	Discharged after	
		2 years	4 years
Individual	6	3	3
Milieu	6	4	3
Rehabilitation	12	4	8

accessible to dynamic psychotherapy, insight oriented or supportive. Drug treatment is a necessary condition for successful psychosocial therapy. However, crises should be worked through and abreacted in the same way as in other patients and not suppressed with drugs.

Comments. This was an ambitious attempt to apply the principles of the scientific experiment to the treatment of chronic schizophrenia. The rehabilitation controls were not allocated at random as were the individual and milieu treatment groups. Since the rehabilitation controls were a prognostically more favourable group, the fact that there were about as many discharges in the two treatment groups indicated that the psychotherapy had been effective. There was no difference in outcome between individual and milieu treatment. However, the groups were too small to allow definite conclusions.

Turku Project (Alanen et al. 1980, 1982–1984)

Theory. A multifacted concept of schizophrenia with emphasis on the interactional origin and psychologically comprehensible nature of the disorder. Psychotherapy was given within the framework of community psychiatry. The outcome was studied with regard to five dimensions:

1. Clinical symptoms
2. Psychodynamic dimension (intrapsychic, interpersonal)
3. Psychosocial dimension (adjustment in work and leisure time, frequency and length of hospital stays)
4. Socioeconomic dimension (sick-leave compensation, disability pension, social assistance)
5. Phenomenological dimension (experience of the disorder and its treatment of patient and relatives).

The approach was problem-oriented as opposed to the "method oriented" approach of which May (1968) is an exponent. Alanen et al. argued that method-oriented research does not do justice to the possibilities of psychotherapeutic activities because an unselected group of schizophrenic patients is heterogeneous from a diagnostic and psychodynamic point of view. Therefore, the treatment, especially psychotherapy, should be individually planned, taking into consideration the nature of the disorder and the patient, including significant interpersonal relationships.

Treatment. Patients were offered a variety of psychotherapeutic treatments, often in combination. Out of 100 schizophrenic patients, 33 received intensive individual therapy (at least once a week for at least 6 months) and 23 infrequent individual therapy (at least once a month).

Patients. Fifty-six patients belonged to the diagnostic group schizophrenia, 10 to schizophreniform psychosis, 14 to schizoaffective psychosis and 20 to borderline psychosis. About three-quarters were hospital cases from the beginning and one-quarter were in open care. The highest daily dose of antipsychotic drugs (corresponding to chlorpromazine) was above 300 mg in 46 patients and

100–300 mg in 46 patients. The average daily dose during the follow-up period was above 100 mg in 22 patients and below in 78. Fifty-two patients only used neuroleptic drugs for brief periods.

Outcome. Outcome was rated both by the therapists and by an independent investigator. On the whole, there was agreement between the raters. In the schizophrenic group about 40% had no psychotic symptoms after 2 years. However, normal working ability was attained in less than 30%, which probably partly reflects unemployment in Finland at that time.

When investigating the therapeutic mechanism of action a positive correlation was found between the patient being referred for psychotherapy and him or her having psychotic symptoms. There was also a positive correlation with working ability, which indicated that psychotherapy was more often given to less severe cases. Intensive individual psychotherapy correlated with psychotic symptoms and several variables which indicated a less severe disorder. On the other hand, the extent of drug therapy was negatively correlated with most prognostic variables. As the authors pointed out, this is a trivial finding since the amount of drug therapy was greatest in the most severe disorders.

Which treatments were actually given out of the total repertoir was not random. Patients with psychological mindedness and capacity for depression got the most intensive psychotherapy, which was also the case with the less autistic patients and those with the lowest degree of symbiotic relations. General intelligence was unrelated to the intensity of psychotherapy.

Authors' Conclusions. The authors claimed that their findings very clearly pointed to the favourable effect of psychotherapy and that they ran counter to the views of May and others that drug treatment is superior to psychotherapy. They argued that a psychotherapeutic attitude is necessary in the treatment and that the genesis, current state and the nature of the interpersonal relationships are mutually interdependent. Care must be devoted to the psychosocial and occupational rehabilitation.

Comments. The study was quasi-experimental. Since the patients were not randomized but allocated to the different treatment modalities according to their respective accessibilities, no conclusions can be drawn concerning the relative merits of the treatment modalities. There was positive selection of cases suitable for intensive psychotherapy as well as a negative selection for intensive drug therapy. Since drugs were given in nearly all cases, albeit in small doses, the low appreciation of drug effects may reflect the authors' attitude more than their actual effects. It does not seem possible to make valid comparisons *within* this material.

On the other hand, the authors intend to make comparisons with previous treatment series where the psychotherapeutic treatment orientation was still under development and the approach therefore probably more traditional. If no great changes have occurred in Finnish society or among Finnish schizophrenic patients during these years, such comparisons may elucidate the significance of psychotherapeutic measures in the treatment of schizophrenic disorders.

Säter Project (Sjöström 1985)

Theory. Basically the theory was psychodynamic with emphasis on object relations. Unfavourable conditions for mental growth during childhood were held to have created an inhibition of emotional development. Classical schizophrenic symptoms such as splitting, catatonia, hallucinations and regression were seen as security measures to reduce anxiety and prevent complete breakdown of the personality. The goal of the therapy was to promote emotional maturation by helping the patient to create as accurate a picture of reality as possible. To that end the psychotherapeutic sessions were concentrated in the more reparative and less regressive phases of the disorder. Close cooperation between the psychotherapist and the ward personnel was fundamental. Drugs were given during phases of excitement, anxiety and tension.

Treatment. One psychotherapist (B. Sandin) treated 14 patients. They were all in the same milieu-treatment-oriented ward. The number of treatment sessions over 8 years varied from 35 to 580, mean 203. Eight of the 14 patients have ended therapy, four are still in therapy, and two have committed suicide.

Patients. All were men, aged 18–28 years, nine fulfilling DSM-III criteria for schizophrenia and five for schizophreniform disorder.

Controls. Twelve male schizophrenic patients were chosen retrospectively from other wards in the same hospital and matched with regard to sex, age ±3 years, diagnosis, treatment during the same time, similar total previous hospitalization and similar working capacity in the preceding year. The controls had received conventional treatment.

Outcome. After 6 years there was a significantly better outcome in the psychotherapy group with regard to time in hospital, employment, symptoms and total outcome score. The rated symptoms were usually less severe but significantly so for only one symptom. The mean dose of antipsychotic drugs during the year preceding the evaluation was far lower (25 mg against 400 mg). Seven out of 12 psychotherapy patients and one out of 12 controls were not prescribed any antipsychotic drugs at all. After 8 years the differences were still greater. The total time in hospital was not significantly different, 290 months versus 427 months for the controls. However, it showed a different distribution, with longer periods during the earlier years and shorter periods during the later years among the psychotherapy patients than among the controls.

Author's Conclusions. The author was cautious due to possible flaws in a retrospective design. He considered, however, the results encouraging enough to motivate further, prospective studies. Individual psychotherapy and milieu treatment both seemed to be necessary for an optimal effect. The fact that the psychotherapy patients spent less and less time in hospital and needed less and less antipsychotic drugs may be seen as a long-lasting effect of the psychotherapy.

Comments. Even though the psychotherapy patients were carefully matched with controls in several prognostically important variables, they were originally selected on the basis of their accessibility to psychotherapy. Therefore, it is difficult to exclude the possibility that right from the start the psychotherapy patients represented a prognostically more favourable group. Therefore, no definite conclusions can be drawn.

General Conclusion

So far there is no Nordic study on the effect of individual psychotherapy in schizophrenia that fulfils all the requirements for a controlled experimental study free from objections. However, the results from all three studies reviewed indicate that psychotherapy together with pharmacotherapy has more favourable effects than each treatment alone. The results form a good basis for prospective studies which are currently under way.

References

Alanen YO, Räkköläinen V, Laakso J, Rasimus R (1980) Problems inherent in the study of psychotherapy of psychoses. Conclusions from a community psychiatric action. Research study. In: Strauss JS, Bowers M, Downey TW, Fleck S, Jackson S, Levine I (eds) The psychotherapy of schizophrenia. Plenum, New York, pp 115–129

Alanen YO, Räkköläinen V, Rasimus R, Laasko J, Järvi R (1982) Developing the treatment of schizophrenia in a community-psychiatric setting. A psychotherapeutic and family-centered approach. Psychiatr Fennica 101–120

Alanen YO, Räkköläinen V, Laakso J, Rasimus R, Järvi R (1983) Psychotherapy of schizophrenia in community psychiatry. 2-year follow-up findings and the influence of selective processes on psychotherapeutic treatments. In: Stierlin H, Wynne LC, Wirsching M (eds) Psychosocial intervention in schizophrenia. Springer, Berlin Heidelberg New York Toronto, pp 67–82

Alanen YO, Räkköläinen V, Rasimus R, Laakso J, Kaljonen A (1984) Psychotherapeutically oriented treatment of schizophrenia: results of 5-year follow-up. In: WPA Regional Symposium, Helsinki, 18–21 June, 1984

Alström JE, Nordlund CL, Persson G (1983) A rating scale for phobic disorders. Acta Psychiatr Scand 68:111–116

Alström JE; Nordlund CL, Persson G, Hårding M, Ljungqvist C (1984a) Effects of four treatment methods on agoraphobic women not suitable for insight-oriented psychotherapy. Acta Psychiatr Scand 70:1–17

Alström JE, Nordlund CL, Persson G, Hårding M, Ljungqvist C (1984b) Effects of four treatment methods on social phobic patients not suitable for insight-oriented psychotherapy. Acta Psychiatr Scand 70:97–110

Alström JE, Nordlund CL, Persson G, Ljungqvist C (1984c) Effects of three non-insight-oriented treatment methods on agoraphobic women suitable for insight-oriented psychotherapy. Acta Psychiatr Scand 70:18–27

Götestam KG, Melin L (1980) A behavioral approach to drug abuse. Drug Alcohol Depend 5:5–25

May RPA (1968) Treatment of schizophrenia. Science House, New York

Öst L-E, Melin L, Götestam KG (1976) A token economy program for chronic schizophrenic patients. Scand J Psychol 17:272–282

Persson G (1984) Early interpersonal relations: experience of four treatment methods in phobic women. Acta Psychiatr Scand 70:111–118

Persson G, Alström JE (1983) A scale for rating suitability for insight-oriented psychotherapy. Acta Psychiatr Scand 68:117–125

Persson G, Alström JE (1984a) Suitability for insight-oriented psychotherapy as a prognostic factor in treatment of phobic women. Acta Psychiatr Scand 69:318–326

Persson G, Alström JE (1984b) Relation between outcome and the patient's initial experience of the therapist and therapeutic conditions in four treatment methods for phobic disorders. Acta Psychiatr Scand 69:296–306

Persson G, Nordlund CL (1983) Expectations of improvement and attitudes to treatment processes in relation to outcome with four treatment methods for phobic disorders. Acta Psychiatr Scand 68:484–493

Persson G, Nordlund CL (1985) Agoraphobics and social phobics: differences in background factors, syndrome profiles and therapeutic response. Acta Psychiatr Scand 71:148–159

Persson G, Alström JE; Nordlund CL (1984) Prognostic factors with four treatment methods for phobic disorders. Acta Psychiatr Scand 69:307–318

Sjödin I (1983) Psychotherapy in peptic ulcer disease. A controlled outcome study. Acta Psychiatr Scand Suppl 307:67

Sjöström R (1985) Effects of psychotherapy in schizophrenia. Acta Psychiatr Scand 71:513–522

Svedlund J (1983) Psychotherapy in irritable bowel syndrome. A controlled outcome study. Acta Psychiatr Scand Suppl 203:67

Uglestad E (1978) Psykotiske langtidspasienter i psykiatriske sykehus – nye behandlingsforsök. Universitetsforlaget, Oslo

Vaglum P, Fossheim I (1980) Differential treatment of young abusers: a quasi-experimental study of a "therapeutic community" in a psychiatric hospital. J Drug Issues 505–515

An Empirical Study of Different Aftercare Strategies for Patients Who Attempted Suicide: The Effect of Psychotherapy on Compliance and Outcome

H.-J. MÖLLER[1], F. BÜRK, A. KURZ, A. TORHORST, C. WÄCHTLER, and H. LAUTER

The results of evaluative research on the prevention of suicidal behaviour are in general rather controversial and inconclusive. There is considerable disagreement, especially over the issue of whether suicidal behaviour can be effectively prevented. In some of the controlled studies a decrease of suicides and suicidal attempts or an improvement of psychopathological disturbances and social maladjustments have been reported. However, the question remains open as to the number of suicide attempters for whom a psychotherapeutic aftercare would seem to be indicated. Another important problem in the aftercare of patients who have attempted suicide is the high rate of non-compliance (Möller and Geiger 1981; Kurz and Möller 1982a, b, 1984a).

Doctors of our psychiatric department are concerned with the psychiatric care of patients who are admitted, after attempted suicide by poisoning, to the Toxicology Department of the Klinikum rechts der Isar, a large general hospital in Munich. This cooperation follows the rules of a psychiatric liaison service (Lauter 1982).

To increase the knowledge of psychotherapeutic aftercare treatment for patients who attempted suicide, we performed a controlled study. Among others, we addressed the following issues:

1. How many patients who are admitted to a general hospital after a suicide attempt require short-therm out-patient psychotherapy in addition to the immediate crisis intervention?
2. Is it possible to increase the aftercare compliance by motivational efforts?
3. Can the compliance be increased by providing continuity of care (i. e. immediate crisis intervention in the hospital and subsequent out-patient treatment offered by the same therapist)?
4. Is a therapeutic management which includes motivational efforts and continuity of care more effective in terms of 1-year outcome than the routine procedure without such characteristics?

The patients were selected from a sample of about 500 patients who were admitted to the Toxicology Department of the Klinikum rechts der Isar. They had all attempted suicide by self-poisoning. The sociodemographic characteristics of this sample deviated from the corresponding data on the general pop-

[1] Psychiatrische Klinik der Technischen Universität Rechts der Isar, Ismaninger Straße 22, D-8000 München 80

Psychological Treatment of Mental Illness
Edited by R. J. Daly and E. A. Sand

Table 1. Sociodemographic data of the original sample ($n=485$) in comparison with the population of Munich

	Patient sample		Population		
	n	%	n	%	
Age					
15–19	82	17	101000	8	$P<0.001$
20–39	275	57	455000	35	
40–59	95	19	328000	25	
60	33	7	257000	20	
Sex					
Male	190	39	547000	48	$P<0.001$
Female	295	61	594000	52	
Marital status					
Single	248	51	543000	48	$P<0.001$
Married	164	34	604000	46	
Divorced	57	12	75000	6	
Widowed	16	3	102000	8	
Unemployment					
Unemployed	80	18	39000	4	$P<0.001$
Employed[a]	372	82	884000	96	

[a] Applied to the age group below 60 years.

ulation of Munich in several important respects (Table 1). Young people females, divorces and unemployed people were overrepresented among the patients. This pattern is well known from previous studies of suicide attempters (Möller et al. 1978). The most frequent psychiatric diagnoses were neurosis, reactive disorder, personality disorder and addictive behaviour (Table 2). Of the patients, 26% reported at least one previous suicidal episode. Regarding sex, age, marital status, previous suicide attempts, psychiatric diagnosis etc., the sample was found to be representative of suicide attempters in general (Möller et al. 1978; Kockott et al. 1970; Kreitman 1977).

Because of the specific limitations of a short-term psychotherapy for suicide attempters on an outpatient basis, about 50% of the original sample could not be included in the aftercare study (Table 3). For only 226 patients did short-term psychotherapeutic aftercare seem to be indicated (Möller et al. 1983).

During the whole research programme the patients of the original sample were randomly assigned to the four collaborating doctors. The research programme was divided into two separate stages. In the first stage the compliance and 1-year outcome of the standard care were studied. In the second stage the effects of motivational efforts and of continuity of care on compliance and 1-year outcome were analysed. The standard care was an immediate crisis intervention in the hospital (with a mean of three sessions) and subsequent referral to special suicide prevention services (Fig. 1). The patients were urged to make

Table 2. Diagnostic distribution of the total sample ($n=485$)

Diagnosis	ICD No.	*n*	%
Psychoses	290–299	57	12
Exogenous	290–294	8	2
Schizophrenic	295	27	6
Affective	296	22	4
Neuroses	300.0	111	23
Depressive	300.4	91	19
Other	300.0, 300.1, 300.5, 300.7	20	4
Personality disorders	301.0	54	11
Hysteric	301.5	17	4
Asthenic	301.6	10	2
Sociopathic	301.7	8	2
Other	301.0, 301.1, 301.2, 301.3, 301.8	19	4
Misuse/addiction	303–305	90	19
Alcohol	303, 305.0	51	10
Drugs	304, 305.5, 305.9	39	8
Reactive and adjustment disorders	308, 309	154	32
Reactive disorders	308	5	1
Adjustment disorders	309	149	31
Other diagnoses		19	4

Table 3. Patients fulfilling exclusion criteria ($n=259$)

	n	%
Drug overdose in addicts (no suicidal intention)	26	10
Psychoses	59	23
Current psychotherapy	44	17
Severe non-psychotic disturbances requiring in-patient treatment	35	14
Poor command of german	19	7
Place of residence outside of Munich area	35	14
No indication for aftercare	21	8
Other reasons	20	8

appointments with these institutions in order to improve compliance. The therapy in these institutions was out of our control. In most of them a psychodynamic approach was practised. In the second stage of the study we directed our attention to the effects of increased motivational efforts. A self-rating questionnaire was given to the patients to obtain a comparable measure of the motivation towards psychotherapy. On the basis of this information, an additional interview was conducted (up to half an hour) centring on motivational deficits (e.g. prejudices and reservations). In addition, the patients received a

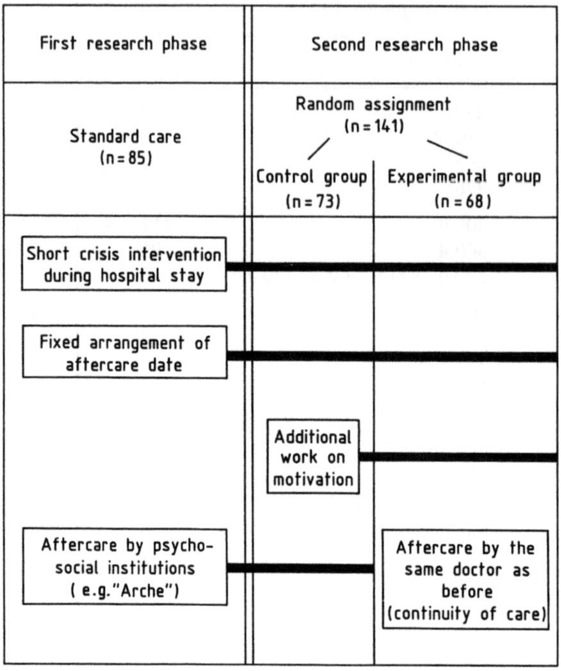

Fig. 1. Design of the study

motivating letter from the doctor to ensure that they accepted the aftercare recommended.

In this second stage, the patients were randomly assigned to two groups: the patients of the experimental group ($n=68$) were offered subsequent ambulatory short-term psychotherapy by the clinician who had already been in charge of the patient in the hospital. Three of the four clinicians were well-trained psychotherapists who had been concerned with suicide attempters within the liaison service over a period of 1–3 years. The concept of the aftercare was determined by the psychotherapeutic training of the doctors: two of them represented a psychoanalytic and one a non-directive paradigm of psychotherapy, whilst the fourth doctor worked with his patients on the basis of a brief introduction into some techniques of behaviour therapy (Kurz and Möller 1984b). The therapy was limited to 12 sessions within 3 months of the initial attempt. The management of the control group ($n=73$) was identical to that of the routine group except that the increased motivational efforts were not made.

Standardized rating instruments were used in the initial assessment of psychopathological symptoms, personality traits and social adjustment. The same rating instruments were used at the beginning, during and at the end of the outpatient treatment (but only for the experimental group), as well as in the follow-up examination. Among others, we applied the Inpatient Multidimen-

Table 4. Characteristics of the three treatment groups

	Standard care group		Control group		Experimental group	
	n	%	*n*	%	*n*	%
Age						
15–19	22	26	15	21	10	15
20–39	46	54	42	58	38	56
40–59	16	19	13	18	17	25
60	1	1	3	4	3	4
Sex						
Male	33	39	25	34	27	40
Female	52	61	48	66	41	60
Marital status						
Single	50	59	38	52	28	41
Married	24	30	24	33	24	36
Widowed	2	2	1	1	2	3
Divorced	9	11	10	14	14	21
Unemployment						
Employed	77	91	60	82	59	87
Unemployed	8	9	13	18	9	13
Previous suicidal episodes						
No	63	74	51	70	49	74
Yes	22	26	22	30	17	26
Previous psychiatric treatment (out-patient)						
No	66	78	55	75	52	77
Yes	19	22	18	25	16	24
Previous psychiatric treatment (in-patient)						
No	75	88	70	96	60	88
Yes	10	12	3	4	8	12
Severity of intoxication (Reed)						
0–3	60	71	53	73	52	76
4, 5	7	8	12	16	9	13
No decision	18	21	8	11	7	10
Neurosis	17	20	24	33	27	40
Personality disorder	9	11	11	15	7	10
Misuse/addiction	17	20	11	15	27	40
Reactive disturbance	37	44	27	37	27	40
Others	5	6	–	–	–	–
Parasuicidal intention	57	69	38	53	42	63
Suicidal intention	26	31	34	47	25	37

Deviations of *n* are due to missing data.

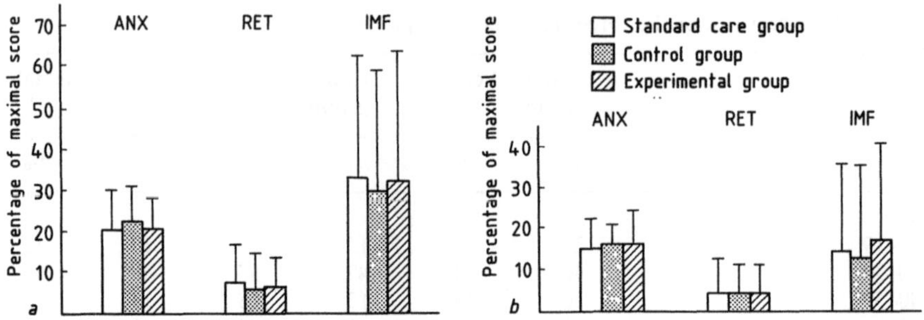

Fig. 2. IMPS Scores on admission (**a**) and at follow-up (**b**). ANX, anxious depression; RET, retardation and apathy; IMF, impaired functioning

sional Psychiatric Rating Scale (IMPS; Lorr 1984), the Depression Self-Rating Scale (DS; v. Zerssen and Koeller 1976), the Social Adjustment Scale (SAS; Weissman and Bothwell 1976), the Freiburger Personality Inventory (FPI; Fahrenberg et al. 1978), the Global Assessment Scale (GAS; Spitzer et al. 1976) and the Drug Taking Evaluation Scale (DTES; Holsten and Waal 1980). In addition to these psychopathometrical data, detailed information was collected on sociodemographical characteristics as well as on the history of psychiatric illness and suicidal behaviour. The outpatient therapy sessions were tape recorded for an analysis of the therapeutic interaction.

No significant differences in sociodemographic characteristics, history of suicidal behavior, history of psychiatric treatment and psychiatric diagnoses were found between the three patient groups (Table 4). Also, the scores of the GAS, IMPS (Fig. 2), FPI; SAS and DS revealed no significant discrepancies between these groups. Thus, it seems meaningful to relate differences of outcome to the different aftercare strategies. However, at present we can only report preliminary results concerning outcome and especially concerning factors probably influencing outcome.

We expected the patients in the control group to display better compliance as a result of motivational efforts. However, the improvement of compliance was small and not significant; the rate of non-compliance is 60% in the routine care group, and 50% in the control group (Table 5). More convincing are the results of the experimental group, showing the effect of continuity of care; only 28% of the patients did not accept the aftercare treatment. Furthermore, the data show that the lower degree of non-compliance in the experimental group is not compensated by higher drop-out rates during aftercare treatment. In fact, 38% of the experimental group remained in therapy for more than five sessions, whereas only 12% of the control group did so.

From this evidence we conclude that continuity of care is an important factor in guaranteeing a high rate of compliance in the aftercare treatment of suicide attempters. The increased motivational efforts, however, were found to be rather ineffective under the conditions tested. In our earlier investigations

Table 5. Compliance of the three treatment groups

Hours of aftercare treatment	Standard care group		Control group		Experimental group	
	n	%	*n*	%	*n*	%
0	51	60	37	50	19	28
1–2	13	15	14	19	11	16
3–5	7	8	13	18	12	18
6–10	5	6	4	6	15	22
>10	6	7	5	7	11	16
Missing data	3	4	0		0	

Experimental group and control group significantly different ($P<0.001$), but standard care group and control group not significantly different.

(Möller and Geiger 1982), the arrangement of a fixed appointment for aftercare proved to be a very important factor for compliance, and additional motivational efforts produced little further increase in the compliance rate.

The patients were followed up 1 year after the initial hospital admission. We were able to collect at least some important data on 90% of the 226 patients. Six patients hat committed suicide, 23 had repeated suicide attempts and there was a total of 49 incidents of recurred suicidal behaviour (suicide and suicidal attempts). Current psychopathological disturbances, measured in various dimensions, were only slightly improved at follow-up when compared with the initial assessment (Fig. 2). This improvement was most obvious for the IMPS factor, "impaired functioning", which reflects unspecific complaints of depressed patients.

To test the efficacy of the different aftercare strategies, we compared the frequency of suicides, suicide attempters, suicide attempts and recurrences of suicidal behaviour between the three groups. The result was notably disappointing, in that the experimental group was significantly ($p<0.05$) worse than the control group with respect to suicidal behaviour (Table 6). The outcome of the experimental group was also a little worse (n.s.) than the outcome of the control group in two other dimensions (rate of psychiatric hospitalization and inability to work) whereas the other outcome criteria (GAS, depression factor of the IMPS, self-rating factor of depression) showed no differences between the groups (Table 7). There were no significant differences concerning 1-year outcome results between the four therapists.

From this evidence, our hypothesis that the patients would benefit more from the experimental aftercare programme than from the routine strategy, has to be reviewed. By combining motivational efforts and continuity of care, we did no better in preventing recurrent suicidal behaviour than by referring the patients to special suicide prevention services. In fact, the routine care programme was superior.

Table 6. Suicidal behaviour during follow-up period

	Standard care group		Control group		Experimental group	
	n	%	*n*	%	*n*	%
Patients with follow-up	82	100	70	100	66	100
Suicide	1	1	2	3	3	5
Suicidal attempt (not before suicide)	11	13	3	4	9	14
Suicidal behaviour	12	15	5	7	12	18
No suicidal behaviour	70	85	65	93	54	82

Experimental group and control group significantly different ($P<0.05$), but standard care group and control group not significantly different.

Table 7. Standardized assessments of outcome of the three treatment groups (figures are mean ± SD)

	Standard care group ($n=80$)	Control group ($n=65$)	Experimental group ($n=62$)
Global assessment scale (GAS)	66.9 ± 14.3	66.9 ± 15.3	65.5 ± 16.8
Anxious depression (IMPS)	12.7 ± 5.7	12.9 ± 5.4	12.9 ± 7.0
Retardation and apathy (IMPS)	3.1 ± 5.6	2.9 ± 4.8	2.8 ± 5.1
Impaired functioning (IMPS)	0.9 ± 1.3	0.9 ± 1.4	1.0 ± 1.5
Depression factor (self-rating)	7.1 ± 7.1	6.2 ± 6.9	7.6 ± 9.2

There are three possible reasons to account for this result:

1. The short-term psychotherapy provided by the four members of our team was not as efficient as the treatment offered by the special suicide prevention services; thus the outcome was worse despite a better compliance
2. The ramdomized location of patients between the experimental and control group was biased. Although the basic social and psychiatric data revealed no significant differences, there is some evidence for an accumulation of risk factors in the experimental group, e.g. being divorced, living alone, duration of unemployment and inability to work in the last 12 months. Thus, outcome in our own patients may have been worse, although the efficacy of standard care and experimental care might be equivalent
3. The influence of the short-term out-patient psychotherapy regarding outcome was minor compared to the effect of the immediate crisis intervention measures in the hospital. This suggestion is supported by the finding that patients who remained in outpatient treatment for two sessions or more did no better than patients who terminated earlier (Table 8). This holds true for all patient groups. Assuming that the impact of the immediate crisis inter-

Table 8. Recidivism of suicidal behaviour related to duration and type of aftercare

	Aftercare		Patients with suicide		Patients with parasuicide		Patients with recurrent suicidal behaviour	
		n	*n*	%	*n*	%	*n*	%
Standard care group	No	51	–	–	6	12	6	12
	Yes	31	1	3	5	16	6	19
	≧3 h	18	–	–	3	17	3	17
Control group	No	37	2	5	1	3	3	8
	Yes	36	–	–	2	6	2	6
	≧3 h	22	–	–	2	9	2	9
Experimental group	No	19	–	–	3	16	3	16
	Yes	49	3	6	6	12	9	18
	≧3 h	38	1	3	6	16	7	18

vention was so dominant in comparison with the additional effect of the outpatient aftercare, the outcome differences between the experimental and control group again must be explained by biased randomization.

Only a more differentiated analysis of the data and the use of more sophisticated procedures, such as multivariate techniques, will enable a final answer to be given.

References

Fahrenberg J, Selg H, Hampel R (1978) Freiburger Persönlichkeitsinventar, FPI. Hogrefe, Göttingen

Holsten F, Waal H (1980) The DTES – Drug taking evaluation scale. A simple scale for the evaluation of drug taking behavior. Acta Psychiatr Scand 61:275–305

Kockott G, Heyse H, Feuerlein W (1970) Der Selbstmordversuch durch Intoxikation. Fortschr Neurol Psychiatr 18:441–465

Kreitman N (ed) (1977) Parasuicide. Wiley, London

Kurz A, Möller H-J (1982a) Ergebnisse der epidemiologischen Evaluation von suizidprophylaktischen Versuchsprogrammen. Psychiatr Prax 9:12–19

Kurz A, Möller H-J (1982b) Ergebnisse der klinisch-experimentellen Evaluation von suizidprophylaktischen Versorgungsprogrammen. Arch Psychiatr Nervenkr 232:97–118

Kurz A, Möller H-J (1984b) Merkmale der psychotherapeutischen Krisenintervention bei Patienten nach Suizidversuch. In: Wolfersdorf M (ed) Depressionsbehandlung in der Klinik. Roderer, Regensburg

Kurz A, Möller H-J (1984a) Hilfesuchverhalten und Compliance von Suizidgefährdeten. Psychiatr Prax 11:6–13

Lauter H (1982) Die pyschiatrische Versorgung von Suizidenten auf internistischen Stationen. In: Fiedler PA, Franke A, Howe J, Kury H, Möller RJ (eds) Herausforderung und Grenzen der klinischen Psychologie. Deutsche Gesellschaft für Verhaltenstherapie, Tübingen

Lorr M (1974) Assessing psychotic behavior by the IMPS. In: Pichot P, Olivier-Martin R (eds) Psychological measurements in psychopharmacology. Karger, Basel (Modern problems in pharmacopsychiatry, vol 7)

Möller H-J, Geiger V (1982) Inanspruchnahme von Nachbetreuungsmaßnahmen durch Parasuizidenten: Probleme und Verbesserungsmöglichkeiten. In: Helmchen H, Linden M, Rüger U (eds) Psychotherapie in der Psychiatrie. Springer, Berlin Heidelberg New York

Möller H-J, Geiger V (1981) Möglichkeiten zur „Compliance"-Verbesserung bei Parasuizidenten. Crisis Int J Suicide Crisis Studies 2:122–129

Möller H-J, Werner V, Feuerlein W (1978) Beschreibung von 150 Patienten mit Selbstmordversuch durch Tabletten – unter besonderer Berücksichtigung des Selbstmordverhaltens und der Inanspruchnahme von Beratungsmöglichkeiten für Suizidgefährdete. Arch Psychiatr Nervenkr 226:113–135

Möller H-J, Bürk F, Kurz A, Torhurst A, Wächtler C, Lauter H (1983) Empirische Untersuchungen zur poststationären Versorgung von Suizidpatienten im Rahmen eines psychiatrischen Liaisondienstes. In: Pohlmeier H, Schmidtke A, Wetz R (eds) Suizidales Verhalten, Methodenprobleme und Erklärungsansätze. Roderer, Regensburg, pp 164–174

Spitzer J, Endicott R-L, Fleiss L (1976) The global assessment scale. A procedure for measuring overall severity of psychiatric disturbances. Arch Gen Psychiatry 33:766–771

Weissman MM, Bothwell S (1976) Assessment of social adjustment by patient self-report. Arch Gen Psychiatry 33:1111–1115

Zerssen D v, Koeller DM (1976) Klinische Selbstbeurteilungs-Skalen (KSb-S) aus dem Münchner Psychiatrischen Informationssystem (PSYCHIS München), Manuale. a) allgemeiner Teil, b) Paranoid-Depressivitäts-Skala, c) Befindlichkeits-Skala, d) Beschwerden-Liste. Beltz, Weinheim

Evaluation of Behaviour Therapy in Anorexia Nervosa

M. M. FICHTER[1] and W. KEESER

Introduction

Almost 300 years ago, long before the terms psychotherapy and anorexia nervosa were coined, Richard Morton (1694) described his therapeutic efforts with an 18-year-old anorexia nervosa patient as follows:

> These Symptoms I did endeavor to relieve by the outward application of Aromatick Bags made to the Region of the Stomach, and by Stomack-Plaisters, as also by the internal use of Bitter Medicines, Chalybeates, and Juleps made of Cephalick and Antihysterick Waters, sufficiently impregnated with Spirit of Salt Aromoniack, and Tincture of Castor, and other things of that Nature. Upon the Use of which she seemed to be much better, but being quickly tired with Medicines, she beg'd that the whole Affair might be committed again to Nature, whereupon consuming every day more and more, she was after three months taken with a Fainting Fit and dyed (Morton 1694, cited in Bliss and Branch 1960, p 11).

Since then anorexia nervosa patients have been treated with a large variety of approaches; somatic treatments include parenteral hyperalimentation (Maloney and Farrell 1980), tube feeding (Williams 1958), pharmacotherapies (Crisp 1965), leucotomy (Crisp and Kalucy 1973), pituitary implantations (Kylin 1937) and electroconvulsive therapy (ECT) (Wall 1959). Psychological treatments of various kinds have been described and advocated, such as psychoanalytic therapy (Gifford et al. 1970), supportive psychotherapy (Farquharson and Hyland 1966), family therapy (Minuchin et al. 1973), dream analysis (Szyrynski 1973), video playback therapy (Gottheil et al. 1969), a psychoeducative approach (Groen and Feldman-Toledano 1966; Cotugno 1980), behaviour therapy following the classical conditioning paradigm (Hallsten 1965; Lang 1965) and behaviour therapy following the operant conditioning paradigm (Agras et al. 1974; Garfinkel et al. 1973; Halmi et al. 1975).

All these treatment procedures have been claimed to be effective. Have we made any progress towards developing effective therapies for anorexia nervosa or is the diversity of treatment approaches for which effectiveness has been claimed just a sign of their futility and the therapist's helplessness when confronted with a patient determined not to eat? These questions bring us right to the core problems of psychotherapy research. The discrepancies between the ideal model of experimental laboratory research design and the realities of psy-

[1] Psychiatrische Klinik und Poliklinik der Universität München, Nußbaumstraße 7, D-8000 München 2, and Psychosomatische Klinik Roseneck, D-8210 Prien

Psychological Treatment of Mental Illness
Edited by R. J. Daly and E. A. Sand

chotherapy research have recently been pointed out in the report of the American Psychiatric Association (APA) commission on methodological and efficacy issues in psychotherapy research (APA 1982, pp 202–203). The following report on behavioural psychotherapy research in anorexia nervosa highlights some research problems which have been encountered in the past (which are not unique for behaviour therapy or anorexia nervosa) and gives some ideas for future research strategies.

Body Weight, Behaviour and Attitude in Anorexia Nervosa

Patients with anorexia nervosa according to the diagnostic criteria of Feighner et al. (1972) who were successive admissions from 1976 to 1978 at the Max-Planck-Institute for Psychiatry (MPI) in Munich were studied in a longitudinal research design. Patients (23 female, 1 male) were studied during in-patient treatment using daily measures of body weight, anorectic attitude and behaviour. The mean age on admission was 19.6 ± 4 years. The patients had had a mean of 1.8 previous inpatient therapies and the mean duration of illness before treatment at the MPI was 3.2 ± 2.4 years). The mean duration of the in-patient therapy programme was 5.0 ± 1.7 months.

Behavioural treatment was conducted in an open psychiatric unit where staff were well trained in the implementation of behaviour therapy. All 24 patients were treated in a broad-spectrum behaviour therapy programme, comparable to that described by Agras and Werne (1977). The treatment was individualized according to each patient's needs and preferences. He or she received incentives such as access to physical and social activities, books, visits to school, or other visiting privileges contingent on daily weight gain. With the exception of severely emaciated patients, a 10-day baseline phase was followed by a non-contingent reinforcement phase; during this phase of treatment goals such as weight gain were set and the patients were verbally encouraged to work towards achieving the goals without backup reinforcement (Agras et al. 1974). This non-contingent programme was sufficient to induce weight gain in only three patients, while a contingent reinforcement programme was implemented in the remaining 21 patients. Figure 1 and Table 1 show the changes in body weight, eating behaviour (nurses' rating) and the self-ratings in the anorexia nervosa inventory for self-rating factor I (figure consciousness), factor IV (adverse effect of meals) and factor VI (bulimia). All these variables showed statistically significant improvement during the course of in-patient therapy (Wilcoxon test for pair differences).

During the baseline phase there was a mean decrease of body weight of 40 g per day ($n = 18$); during the non-contingent reinforcement phase body weight increased by 137 g per day ($n = 12$) and during contingent reinforcement body weight increased by 290 g per day ($n = 17$). This increase was statistically significant when compared with baseline ($p < 0.001$) and with non-contingent reinforcement (two-tailed $P = 1$; median test and Kruskal–Wallis one-way

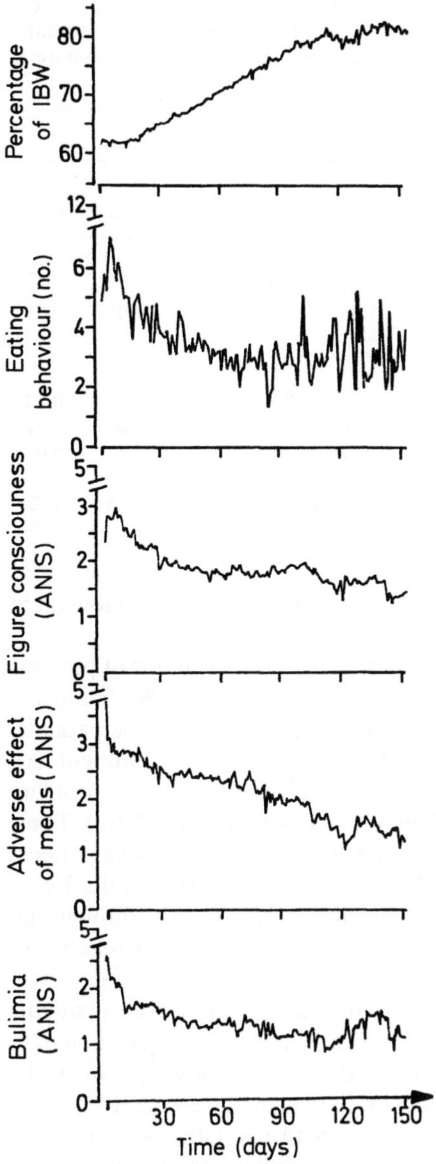

Fig. 1. Daily changes in body weight and factors of the anorexia nervosa inventory for self-rating (ANIS) during the course of in-patient treatment. (Reprinted with permission from Fichter et al. 1982)

analysis of Variance). The major changes of eating behaviour (as rated by the nurses) occurred within the first 6 weeks of treatment and the same applies to the self-rating of figure consciousness and bulimia. Mean body weight increased from 61.2% of ideal body weight (IBW) on admission to 84.4% at discharge, 78.4% at 3-year follow up and 85.9% at 7-year follow up. During the time of hospital treatment all female patients showed amenorrhea; at the 3-

Table 1. Mean ($\bar{x}$) and standard deviations (SD) of body weight and the anorexia nervosa inventory for self-rating (ANIS; factors "figure consciousness", "negative effect of meals" and "bulimia") on admission, after initial (10%) weight gain and at discharge in anorexia nervosa patients

	Admission[a]		Initial weight gain[b]		Discharge[a]		*P* values		
	$\bar{x}$	SD	$\bar{x}$	SD	$\bar{x}$	SD	a vs. b	b vs. c	a vs. c
Weight									
Body weight (kg)	34.9	5.7	41.5	5.6	47.4	1.8			
Body weight (% IBW)	61.2	6.7	75.7	5.3	84.4	6.0	0.01	0.01	0.01
Anis (o–s)									
Total score	2.75	1.0	2.33	1.0	1.29	0.9	0.05	–	0.02
Figure consciousness	3.09	1.3	1.93	1.1	0.88	0.9	0.01	0.05	0.01
Negative effect of meals	2.61	1.2	2.12	1.4	1.10	0.9	–	–	0.02
Bulimia	2.02	1.6	1.53	1.9	0.42	1.0	–	0.05	0.02

year follow up amenorrhea was present in 61% and at the 7-year follow up in 39% of all female patients.

A common problem in psychotherapy research is the drop out of patients during therapy; Pierloot et al. (1982) and Vandereycken et al. (1983) reported a 50% drop-out rate during inpatient treatment of anorexia nervosa patients. In our series there was no apparent drop out during inpatient treatment. All patients were in the unit for at least 3 months. An even more serious problem is the generally low response rate in follow-up assessments (Hsu 1980). Thus, in the study by Pierloot et al. (1982) only 78 of 128 anorexia nervosa patients could be followed up after an average of 4.2 years after discharge. At the 3-year follow up in our study all except one patient and at the 7-year follow up all except two patients were interviewed personally. For these patients reliable information was obtained from close relatives, self-ratings and telephone interview with the patients. Generally, there were indications that several patients had a chronic illness and one patient died in the seventh year after discharge. Except for this fatality, outcome was better at the 7-year follow up than at the 1- or 3-year follow up. At the 7-year follow up the mean body weight was even higher than at discharge (with a higher variance between patients). Only 39% of all female patients had amenorrhea at the 7-year follow up, compared with 61% at the 3-year follow up and 100% at discharge. Our data, collected daily during inpatient treatment, indicate that body weight and specific anorectic behaviours and attitudes showed significant improvement during inpatient treatment, while attitudes of a more general neurotic scope such as the feeling of insufficiency, general distress, (sexual) anxieties and obsessiveness (anancasm) did not. Further evidence of this interpretation is given by the follow up data. While little change was observed in those more general variables assessed during inpatient treatment, scores on admission on the scales of "general distress," "insufficiency" and the factor "emotional lability" of the Freiburger personality inventory were significantly correlated with poor prognosis at the 3-year follow up. Future treatment programmes should therefore include strategies directed at the more general variables, which appear more resistent towards change in present (behaviour) therapy programmes.

Recently the effect of behaviour therapy in anorexia nervosa has been reviewed by Garfinkel and Garner (1980). The main effect of behaviour therapy appears to be in inducing weight gain. Behaviour therapy must be criticized in that it has neglected other dependent variables besides weight gain, and therapies directed towards other behaviours and attitudes should be investigated. Thirteen of the 30 behaviour therapy studies reviewed by Garfinkel and Garner were single-case studies reporting on only one or two patients. They state that several recent studies

> have verified the impressive short-term effects of operant conditioning on weight. However, there has been only one predictive controlled study with randomization of subjects assigned to behavioral or non-behavioural groups (Eckert et al. 1979). This study found no significant differences between behavioural treatment and milieu therapy alone, in terms of weight gain over 35 days. But these results may have been due to the particular operant methodology used, i.e. rewarding every five days (rather than daily as is usually recommended), not individualizing rewards, and only studying the groups for one month (Garfinkel and Garner 1982, p 231).

This multicentre project has been one of the largest studies for therapy evaluation in anorexia nervosa that has so far been conducted. Eighty-one anorexia nervosa patients were randomly assigned to one of four treatment combinations of cyproheptadine or placebo with behaviour therapy or no behaviour therapy. The implementation of large-scale multicentre projects employing group statistics is expensive and the cited study shows how much in vain such efforts can be. The research strategy of group-statistical designs definitely has its limitations in clinical research.

Sidman (1960) has criticized group statistics in that they "obscure both personal performance and transition states." In disorders with low prevalence it is difficult to obtain homogeneous groups of sufficient size. Methodological, practical and ethical problems are brought about by the use of control groups. Due to these unresolved problems single-case experimental designs have been advocated as an alternative (Hersen and Barlow 1976). Together with some new statistical methods, known as ARIMA time-series models, this approach is a powerful methodology for studying outcome and process characteristics.

Treatment evaluation is necessary both from scientific considerations and for clinical implementation. Ideally, such evaluation should take into account the nature of both intervention and the therapeutic change desired in the patient. However, the common evaluation techniques do not take into account the subtleties of the therapeutic process or all of its effects. There is a preference for using repeated measurement designs with rarely more than two time points (classical outcome study with a before-after design), neglecting ongoing processes during treatment and thus the time dimension of change. There is also a predominance of group-statistical analysis, neglecting the pronounced individual differences in response to therapy. Finally, there is a tendency to measure only one dependent variable or to univariately assess treatment effects, neglecting the complexity of the illness and the multiple interactions of change indicators over time.

Apart from measurement issues, methodological refinement in data analysis is necessary for assessing a patient's performance and changes during therapy. A statistical tool meeting such a demand is time-series analysis based on the ARIMA model (Box and Jenkins 1976) which has recently been transferred from econometrics to the social and behavioural sciences (Gottman 1981). The basic approach of time-series analysis is to identify and estimate the underlying stochastic model, which has generated a series of observations. According to Box and Jenkins such a model can be parsimoniously described by its autoregressive (AR) components (i.e. the time-series "remembers" its own past), its moving average (MA) components (i.e. the time-series "remembers" the impact of random shocks having entered the series) or both. If a series does not fluctuate around some fixed mean (i.e. has a trend) it is called non-stationary or integrated (I) and can be differentiated to fulfill the stationarity criterion. Univariate ARIMA models can be used to describe a series and to forecast future behaviour. If more than one time series is involved, there is a distinction between unidirectional influences of one or more stochastic and/or deterministic input series to one output system (i.e. transfer and intervention models), and multidirectional influences of one or more input series to one or more output series (multivariate models). While all models allow causal statements about input–output relationships in that they account for temporal sequences, multivariate models additionally make it possible to detect multiple feedback relationships between all series. In our study with 24 anorexia nervosa patients we have analyzed outcome data in a group-statistical design and in addition we have employed time-series analysis based on the ARIMA model in single cases. The complex mathematical aspects and procedural issues concerning multivariate time series models have been discussed by Tiao and Box (1981) and Jenkins and Alavi (1981). We will restrict ourselves here to a case example to provide information about the applicability and results of interventions in a multivariate time-series analysis.

Case Description

Brigitte, a 19-year-old patient with anorexia nervosa, was treated on an inpatient basis at the MPI for 15 weeks. Two years before anorectic behaviour started, an operation was performed because of an arteriovenous aneurism precentrally located in the right hemisphere. One year after the operation her brother died and the patient suffered from mood disturbances. Later she started to diet and became amenorrhoic. After separation from a boyfriend she attempted suicide and lost further weight. During inpatient treatment she re-

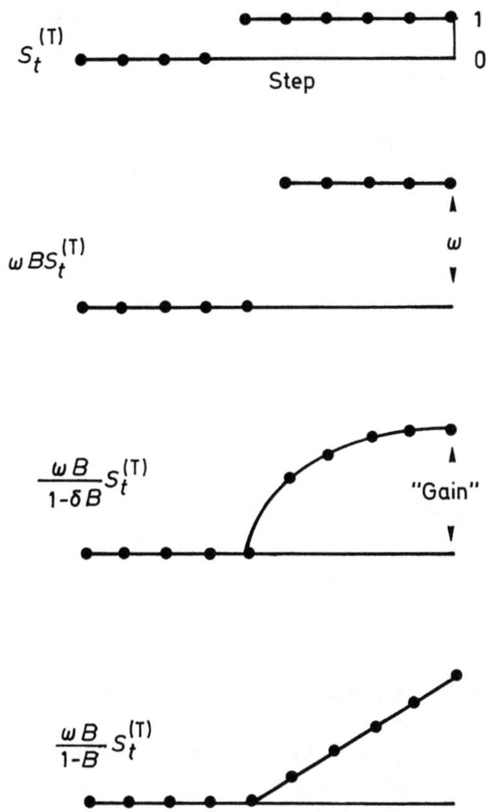

Fig. 2. Possible responses of a time series to an intervention effect. From *top* to *bottom:* example of unitary discrete change; non-dynamic discrete change; dynamic change where speed and "gain" are determined by input lag (ω) and output lag (δ); linear trend

gained weight in the contingent reinforcement phase. Besides body weight, anorectic behaviour and attitudes and the general feeling of wellbeing were measured daily.

Time-Series Analysis. To assess the dynamics of the change process, time-series analyses were performed, using the daily measured weight and self-ratings in the anorexia nervosa inventory (Fichter and Keeser 1980) and the *Befindlichkeitsskala* (Bf-S) by v. Zerssen (1976) Analysis involved identification and estimation of univariate series including intervention models by the PACK Program (Pack 1983). For identification and estimation of the multivariate time series, the Wisconsin multiple time-Series programs were used (Tiao et al. 1979).

Using a time-series intervention model, a wide variety of intervention effects can be tested. These effects may either represent a dynamic response of the series to an intervention, or the more familiar discrete change in level caused by an intervention (the intervention is mostly coded in a binary form with 1 defining the presence of a specific condition and 0 the absence). Figure 2 shows the most common responses of an output series to a change in the input condition: a non-dynamic discrete change in level; a dynamic change in which the speed and the "gain," i.e. the amount of change to a final level, are determined by the input-lag (ω) and the output-lag parameters (δ); and a linear trend (with $\delta = 1$ and the magnitude of the input effect being identical to a linear slope). On advantage of time-series intervention modelling is its adaptive capacity to find out which of these three models is adequate. Specifying a model

$$Z_t = \frac{\omega_0}{1-\delta B} X_t, \tag{1}$$

where Z_t stands for the measured times series, X_t for the dummy vector of the intervention model consisting of 0 s and 1 s, and the expression

$$\frac{\omega_0}{1-\delta B} \tag{2}$$

is a difference equation with the backshift operator B acting on Z_t in such a way $BZ_t = Z_{t-1}$ (e.g. B lags the times series by the factor of the power of B). Alternatively, Eqn. 2 can be expanded as a Taylor series yielding

$$\omega_0(1+\delta B+\delta^2 B^2+ \ldots \delta'' \mathrm{B}'') \tag{3}$$

The results of the non-linear estimation procedure indicate an intervention effect of type A if the estimated δ is 0 (or very close to 0) and of type C if the estimated δ is 1 (or very close to 1). Testing the significance of the estimated intervention parameters poses a serious statistical problem, since time-series data are usually not independent of each other but autocorrelated. The common group-statistical procedure defining the significance merely as a function of the ratio between treatment variance and error variance cannot be applied for testing, because the necessary condition of error independence is usually violated. Instead, time-series intervention models have three sources of variance: the treatment variance, the variance of the dependency (ARIMA) model, and the error variance. Depending on the form of autocorrelation, any neglect of the dependency-model variance leads to dramatic over- or underestimation of statistical significance (Box 1976). To solve the problem, a three-step procedure has to be used. An ordinary least-squares approach is first applied to eliminate the treatment effect. Using the residuals of the first step the underlying ARIMA model is identified and the full model with the intervention part and the ARIMA part is simultaneously estimated by

$$Z_t = \frac{\omega_0}{1-\delta B} X_t + \frac{\theta_q(B)}{\phi_p(B)} a_t,$$

where

$$\phi_q(B) = 1 - \phi_1 B - \ldots - \phi_q \mathrm{B}^q$$

Table 2. Results of the time-series intervention model

$$Z_t = 36.46 + \frac{0.105}{1-0.978\,B} X_{1,t} + \frac{0.366}{1-0.959\,B} X_{2,t} + \frac{1}{1-0.490\,B-0.248\,B^2}\alpha_t$$

where B is the backshift operator: $BZ_t = Z_{t-1}$
$B^2 Z_t = Z_{t-2}$

$X_{1,t}$: non-contingent reinforcement (day 11–day 49)
$X_{2,t}$: contingent reinforcement (day 50–day 110)

$R^2 = 0.99$ (i.e. 99% of the variance is explained by the model)
"Gain" (incontingent reinforcement): 0.10519/(1−0.97823) = 4.83 kg
"Gain" (contingent reinforcement): 0.36646/(1−0.95862) = 8.86 kg

is the moving average polynom of order q and

$$\theta_p(B) = 1 - \theta_1 B - \ldots - \theta_p B^p$$

is the autoregressive polynom of order p. The a_ts are independently, identically and normally distributed random shocks (or white noise) with zero mean and variance σ^2.

A prerequisite for the above procedure is the specification of the intervention effect in the form of a vector using a binary coding system of 0 and 1. In the case example presented, the effect of the non-contingent reinforcement schedule during day 11 to day 49 of the treatment and the contingent reinforcement schedule during day 50 to day 110 were considered as an intervention.

The identification and estimation of multivariate versus univariate time-series models poses complex problems, for which several partly incompatible solutions have been proposed. One potentially misleading strategy suggests identifying a univariate ARIMA model for every series and assessing the multivariate relationship using the residuals of the univariate ARIMA models (Jenkins and Alavi 1981). The method for identification used in this paper was developed by Tiao and Box (1981). Its main characteristic is the attempt to identify an overall multivariate model directly from the original data. The procedure involves: (1) Inspection of the cross-correlation matrices and the stepwise multivariate autoregressive coefficients of all time series to identify type (multivariate autoregressive and/or moving average) and order of the multivariate ARIMA model, (2) estimation of the identified model and (3) model diagnostics by inspection of the residuals' cross-correlation and stepwise multivariate autoregressive coefficients. Multivariate ARIMA modelling is an empirical, iterative process leading to stepwise emergence of the driving forces of the multivariate process. The final estimated coefficients of the series' interrelationships can be used mathematically and graphically to describe strength and direction of mutual influences and to draw conclusions about causal chains.

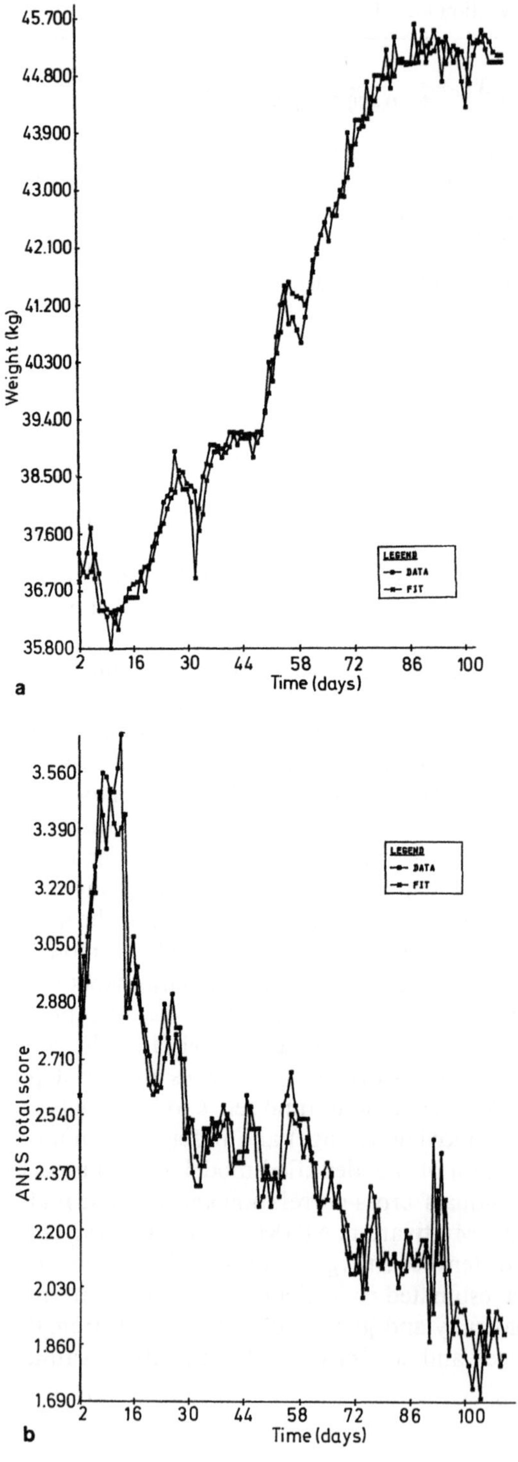

Fig. 3. Real data and fitted values for **a** body weight and **b** ANIS total score (based on intervention and the ARIMA dependency model) for case 50

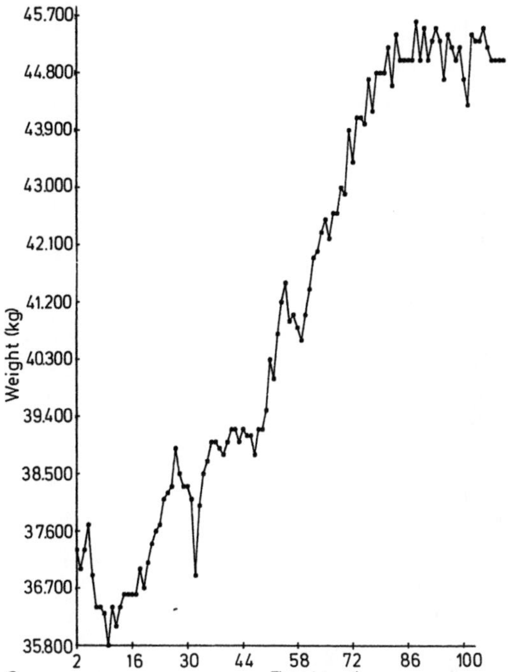

a

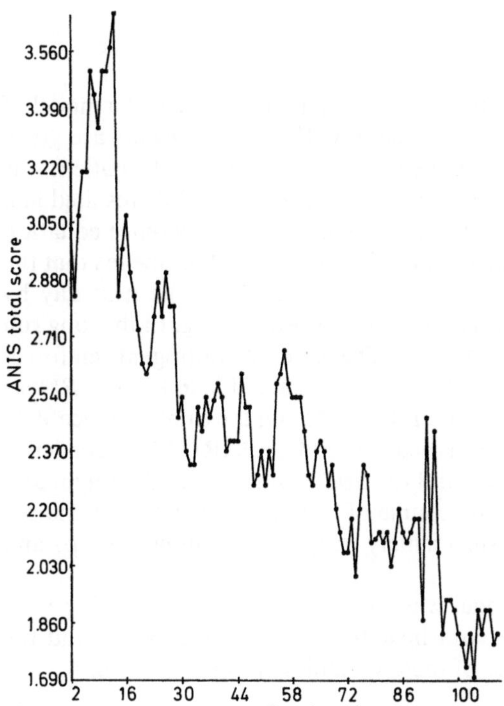

b

Fig. 4 a–c. Data for **a** body weight and **b** ANIS total score and **c** the *Befindlichkeits-Skala* (BfS) over time (in days) for case 50 (Fig. 4c see p. 88)

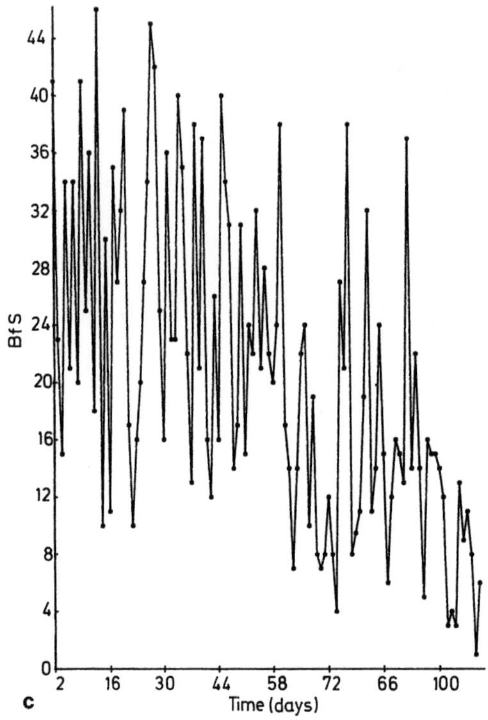

Fig. 4c

Results of Time-Series Analysis. The intervention analysis revealed a model of type B (dynamic change) for both intervention effects. The results are given in Table 2. During the baseline phase the mean body weight of the patient was 36.5 kg. The onset of the non-contingent reinforcement schedule resulted in a dynamic rise of weight; its shape was determined by the difference equation 0.105/1–0.978 *B*, which can be expanded as Taylor series. This means that the first day of intervention increased the weight by 0.105 kg, the next day by 0.105 × 0.978 kg and each further day by $0.105 \times 0.978^{(t-1)}$ kg. In the long run this would result in a final gain of 4.83 kg. The effect of contingent reinforcement was more pronounced, as can be seen from a gain of 8.86 kg. The R^2 was 0.99 and this indicates and excellent fit of the model. Of the total variance 99% was thus explained by both the intervention and the ARIMA dependency model. Figure 3 shows the real data and the fitted values for body weight and for the ANIS total score during the course of treatment of this anorexic patient. As can be seen, the fit is surprisingly adaptive to follow the ups and downs of the weight course.

A multivariate time-series model was calculated with the following variables: body weight, anorexia nervosa inventory (ANIS) total score and the score of the BfS. The time courses of these variables are shown in Fig. 4.

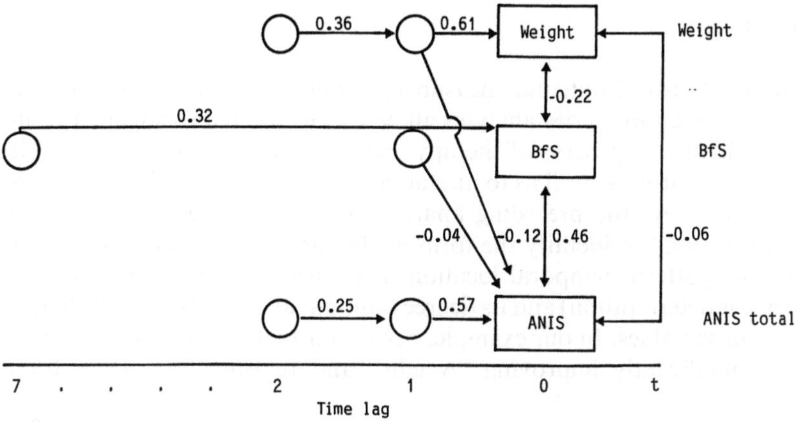

Fig. 5. Pictorial representation of the final ARIMA model derived from the data of case 50 with intercorrelations between variables (weight, *Befindlichkeits-Skala* (BfS) and ANIS total score) with time lag 0–7

The pattern of the cross-correlation matrices of the three variables showed an exponential decay typical for a multivariate autoregressive process. The stepwise multivariate autoregressive matrices were significant at lags 1 and 2 for weight and the ANIS and at lag 7 for the BfS, suggesting multiplicative multivariate autoregressive processes of orders 2 and 7. In such a model 27 ($3 \times 3 \times 3$ variables) autoregressive paths can be estimated. In maximum-likelihood estimation only six paths were significant. The residuals of the final model showed neither significant autocorrelations nor significant cross-correlations. With the residual error correlations, estimates of the "true" synchronous relationship between the five variables were obtained. Figure 5 gives a graphical representation of the final ARIMA model, which consisted of time-delayed (lags 1, 2 and 7) and synchronous (lag 0) components. Weight correlated negatively with mood (i.e. the higher the weight the worse was the mood) and the correlation of mood with ANIS was 0.46. The lagged (delayed) relationships were of interest, particularly that weight was forcing drive at lag 1 for the ANIS total score, which can with some caution be explained in terms of causality for which temporal sequence is a necessary but not sufficient condition. With regard to clinical issues, the model revealed two important findings: (1) changes in body weight affected with a delay of 1 day the subjective component of the anorectic state, as measured by the ANIS questionaire, but have not been the target of any of the measured variables; (2) the ANIS scale mirrored changes in both weight and in mood, which can be seen as a further indicator of the validity of that measurement tool. Thus, the model allows the tentative conclusion regarding the effects of behaviour therapy for this patient, that weight was solely a function of its own past, up to two days. There was no compensating effect, as is often seen with other disorders, where a high value is at least partly compensated by a low value the next day or vice versa.

Discussion

While group-statistical outcome measures provide in overall assessment of a treatment's effect, time-series analyses allow one to subtly investigate, for individual patients, the process of therapy and its effects with regard to single therapeutic indicators as well as to interactions of relevant variables in a multivariate system. As the preceding analysis of a case showed, intervention models can be used to identify the form of the therapeutic effect (discrete vs dynamic), its pattern (temporal location of change and fluctuations of improvement or deterioration) and its degree (amount and significance of change of dependent variables. In our example, behaviour therapy appeared to be effective in significantly improving "weight" and reducing the ANIS total score.

Multivariate times-series analyses were found to be a promising tool for understanding the therapeutic processes. They allow one to assess mutual influences in terms of their temporal relationships and thus to identify leading variables for the therapeutic success or failure. One clinically important outcome of the case example analyzed was the emergence of complex interwoven synchronous and lagged relationships between the measured variables. It allowed one to look into an individual's multidimensional "anorexia system" and to detect the main paths determining the dynamics of that system. A major shortcoming in the design of the case study presented concerns the unavailability of multiple time-series data before and after treatment. Such data would have allowed additionally the estimation of a multivariate ARIMA model for the baseline and the follow up conditions and to compare the dynamic structures operating before, during and after therapy. The study of a multivariate baseline anorexia system might foster an individual tailoring of a therapeutic regimen concentrating on specific illness-producing and maintaining variables. The comparison of these systems before and after treatment can enhance knowledge of the therapeutic effects for an individual patient. In terms of research, the advantage of the idiographic strategy is its ability to detect time patterns of anorexia nervosa for different patients, which would have gone unrecognized with a group-statistical approach. The results of single-subject time-series analyses can be aggregated, processed via classical group-statistical methods (e.g. cluster analysis, uni- and/or multivariate analysis of variance) and used empirically to form nomothetical statements.

References

American Psychiatric Association Commission on Psychotherapy (1982) Methodological and efficacy issues. In: American Psychiatric Association (ed) Psychotherapy Research. Washington, D.C.

Agras S, Werne J (1977) Behavior modification in anorexia nervosa. In: Vigersky RA (ed) Anorexia nervosa. Raven, New York

Agras S, Barlow DH, Chapin HN, Abel GG, Leitenberg H (1974) Behavior modification of anorexia nervosa. Arch Gen Psychiatry 30:279–286

Bliss EL, Branch CHH (1960) Anorexia nervosa. Its history, psychology, and biology. Hoeber, New York

Box GEP (1976) Science and statistics. J Am Stat Ass 71:791–799

Box GEP, Jenkins GM (1976) Time-series analysis: forecasting and control, rev ed. Holden Day, San Francisco

Gifford S, Murawski BJ, Pilot ML (1970) Anorexia nervosa in one of identical twins. Int Psychiatr Clin 7:139–228

Cotugno AJ (1980) A psychoeducational approach in the treatment of anorexia nervosa. Psychol Schools 17:222–240

Crisp AH (1965) Clinical and therapeutic aspects of anorexia nervosa – a study of thirty cases. J Psychosom Res 9:67–78

Crisp AH, Kalucy RS (1973) The effect of leucotomy in intractable adolescent weight phobia (primary anorexia nervosa). Postgrad Med J 49:833–893

Eckert ED, Goldberg SC, Halmi KA et al. (1979) Alcoholism in anorexia nervosa. In: Pickens R, Heston L (eds) Psychiatric factors in drug abuse. Grune & Stratton, San Francisco

Eckert ED, Goldberg SC, Halmi KA, Casper RC, Davis JM (1979) Behavior therapy in anorexia nervosa. Br J Psychiatry 134:55–59

Farquharson RF, Hyland HH (1938) Anorexia nervosa. Metabolic disorder of psychologic origin. JAMA 111:1085–1092

Farquharson RF, Hyland HH (1966) Anorexia nervosa: The course of 15 patients treated from 20 to 30 years previously. Cor Med Ass J 94:9

Feighner JP, Robins E, Guze SB, Woodruff RA, Winokur G, Munoz R (1972) Diagnostic criteria for use in psychiatric research. Arch Gen Psychiatry 26:57–63

Fichter MM, Keeser W (1980) Das Anorexia Nervosa Inventar zur Selbstbeurteilung (ANIS). Arch Psychiatr Nervenkr, 228:67–89

Fichter MM, Doerr P, Pirke KM, Lund R (1982) Behavior attitude, nutrition and endocrinology in anorexia nervosa. Acta Psychiatr Scand 66:429–444

Garfinkel PE, Garner D (1980) Anorexia nervosa. Bruner and Marcel, New York

Garfinkel PE, Kline SA, Stancer HC (1973) Treatment of anorexia nervosa using operant conditioning techniques. J Nerv Ment Dis 157:428–433

Gottheil E, Backup CE, Cornelison FS Jr (1969) Denial and self-image confrontation in a case of anorexia nervosa. J Nerv Ment Dis 148:238–250

Gottmann JM (1981) Time-series analysis. A comprehensive introduction for social scientists. Cambridge University Press, Cambridge

Groen JJ, Feldman-Toledano Z (1966) Educative treatment of patients and parents in anorexia nervosa. Br J Psychiatry 112:671–181

Hallsten EA Jr (1965) Adolescent anorexia nervosa treated by desensitization. Behav Res Ther 3:87–91

Halmi KA, Powers P, Cunningham S (1975) Treatment of anorexia nervosa with behavior modification. Arch Gen Psychiatry 32:93–96

Hersen M, Barlow D (1976) Single-case experimental designs: strategies for studying behaviour change. Pergamon, Oxford

Hsu LKG (1980) Outcome of anorexia nervosa. Arch Gen Psychiatry 37:1041–1046

Jenkins GM, Alavi AS (1981) Some aspects of modelling and forecasting multivariate time series. J Time Series Anal 2:1–47

Kylin R (1937) Magersucht in der weiblichen Spätpubertät. Dtsch Arch Klin Med 180:115–152

Lang P (1965) Behaviour therapy with a case of anorexia nervosa. In: Ullmann LP, Krasner L (eds) Case studies in Behaviour Modification. Holt, Rinehardt, Winston, New York

Maloney MJ, Farrell MK (1980) Treatment of severe weight loss in anorexia nervosa with hyperalimentation and psychotherapy. Am J Psychiatry 137:310–314

Minuchin S, Baker L, Liebmann R, Milman L, Rosmann B, Todd T (1973) Anorexia nervosa: successful application of a family therapy approach. Pediatr Res 7:294
Morton R (1960) Phthisiologica – or a Treatise of Consumption. In: Bliss EL, Branch CHH (eds) Anorexia nervosa. Hoeber, New York, pp 10–11
Pack DJ (1983) The PACK SYSTEM User's Guide. Automatic Forecasting Systems, Hatboro, Pennsylvania
Pierloot R, Vandereycken W, Verhaest S (1982) An inpatient treatment program for anorexia nervosa patients. Acta Psychiatr Scand 66:1–8
Sidman M (1960) Scientific research. Evaluating experimental data in psychology. Basic, New York
Szyrynski V (1973) Anorexia nervosa and psychotherapy. Am J Psychother 27:492–505
Tiao GC, Box GEP (1981) Modeling multiple time series with applications. Am Stat Ass 76:802–816
Tiao GC, Box GEP, Grupe MR, Hudak GB, Bell WR, Chang I (1979) The Wisconson multiple time series program. A preliminary guide. University of Wisconsin, Department of Statistics, Madison
Vandereycken W, Pierloot R (1983) Drop-out during in-patient treatment of anorexia nervosa. A clinical study of 133 patients. Br J Med Psychol 56:145–156
Wall JH (1959) Diagnosis, treatment and results in anorexia nervosa. Am J Psychiatry 115:997–1001
Williams W (1958) Anorexia nervosa: a somatic disorder. Br Med J 2:190–195
Zerssen DV, Koeller DM (1976) Klinische Selbstbeurteilungen aus dem Münchner Psychiatrischen Informationssystem. Beltz, Weinheim

Evaluation of Psychological Treatments for Depression

P. HERMANN[1]

Introduction

The purpose of this paper is to discuss some of the methodological problems in the evaluation of psychological treatments of depressive states. Most of the problems I shall discuss are not specific to the field of depressive states and may be encountered in any evaluation of psychiatric treatment (Cronholm and Daly 1983), especially in psychotherapy research. However, they often present some particular aspects in the field of psychological treatments of depressive states.

There are some prerequisites that concern all psychotherapy research methodologies. The methods or the instruments employed in research must fulfill the following requirements: (a) they must give a usable image of the objects they claim to represent (validity), and (b) they must be able to evaluate or measure the object in a stable, reproducible way (reliability). In addition, they must be acceptable to the clinicians who will accept or reject our research protocols. This means that any attempts to prove the adequacy of our hypothesis should not interfere with or bias the practice we want to study.

Depressive states are frequent (Sartorius 1975). They are often treated by psychotherapy (Arieti and Bemporad 1980; Haynal 1983; Schneider 1978) with or without psychotropic drugs. In spite of this, there are relatively few studies of the effects of psychological treatments on these illnesses (Seligman et al. 1976). As Klerman et al. (1974) wrote: "Relatively few, if any, systematic attempts have been made to study psychotherapy in depressed patients." Lambert (1979) cites a number of studies, but they are based on several different theoretical backgrounds and it is not obvious that they are comparable as far as the results of the treatment are concerned. The methodologies differ according to the different theoretical frameworks. For example, psychotherapy analogues may be acceptable to some schools, but are rejected by others (Gerin 1984). This means that studies that are meaningful for some schools of thought are not acceptable to others because of requirements related to their theoretical frameworks.

Since 1977 a number of papers have been published on the subject of treatment of depression. The reviews by Weissman (1979), Whitehead (1979), and

[1] Unit for Clinical Investigation, University Psychiatric Institutions, 6–8 rue du XXXI-Décembre, CH-1207 Genève

Psychological Treatment of Mental Illness
Edited by R. J. Daly and E. A. Sand

Akiskal (1983) are especially notable. The majority of the papers are concerned with the results of behavioural and cognitive-behavioural therapies (Rehm and Kornblith 1979; Becker and Schuckit 1978; Taylor and Marshall 1977). The fact that there are more controlled studies referring to behavioural or cognitive-behavioural doctrines than to psychoanalytic doctrines may stem from the degree of emphasis on the relationship between therapist and patient, or on the therapeutic use of this relation, which seems to differ between these schools. This has methodological consequences: behavioural or cognitive protocols are easier to standardize and seem to provoke fewer reservations from the clinicians who use these methods.

Depressive states are not only frequent, they are often serious. We are well aware of the severity of the evolution of certain depressive states, either towards, chronicity or towards death, particularly by suicide but probably also in other ways such as somatic disease (Schmale 1958; Schmale and Iker 1965, 1971).

Any clinical decision is uncertain (Hermann 1984), and every decision taken obliges the clinician to choose between risks. One would expect that the clinician would take less risks in depressive states, and introduce the criterion of least regret when choosing treatment strategies, making the decision which, if it proves wrong, would result in the least damage. In any case, clinical decision making is especially important in depressive states (Keller et al. 1982) and must be taken into consideration in study designs. As a general rule research protocols should not interfere, or at least interfere minimally, with clinicians' spontaneous decision-making process. This is not only for the sake of the patients or the patient–clinician relationship, but also for the sake of the research results. We can always train clinicians to do things to meet the requirements of research design, but we should then realize that what we receive at the end is no longer meaningful for the treatment we wanted to study, only for the analogue we have substituted. In other words, we have changed the very object we want to study. In fact there are two conflicting attitudes here that must not be confounded. It has been maintained that each therapeutic decision is an experiment. The researcher may consider each therapeutic decision as an experiment since what he or she values is the information which will allow the confirmation or refutation of the hypothesis. The clinician, on the other hand, uses theories as an aid in the decision-making process, as a tool to help make predictions. He or she uses these predictions to make therapeutic choices in order to get the desired positive results. While the researcher is centred on the information, the clinician is centred on the patient. The researcher wants to prove something, and both positive and negative results are of interest insofar as they allow refutation or confirmation of the hypothesis. The researcher works within the context of justification. In addition to the context of justification, Reichenbach (1938) described the context of discovery, which is to some extent the opposite of the former. He considered that what he called the context of discovery did not need to be explained, despite the fact that the process of discovery is far from clear (Holton 1973, 1978; Hermann and Tricot 1984). We may add yet another context, that of application, which is the field of any practician or clinician who uses predictions founded on the chosen theories to make therapeutic choices in order to get the desired result for the patient. These different attitudes, discovery, justification, and application, are often difficult to distinguish and can result in confusion. They reflect different projects and although they are incompatible at any one time, in the long term they are necessary complementary steps in the acquisition of knowledge.

Some clinical and methodological consequences result:

In population studies the more rigourous the research protocol, the less flexible it will be, and the greater the number of unusable cases will be (especially from drop-outs). This not only increases the size of the initial sample necessary, but also introduces selection of cases: only the patients who have accepted the protocol of that particular research can be included. This touches on the question of patient motivation, and a number of studies have shown that this factor is of importance (Gomes-Schwartz 1978; Keithly et al. 1980; Gerin 1984).

The sample population may be biased, since the clinician will avoid exposing patients considered most likely to be harmed by additional risk. The clinician might also, somewhat paradoxically, hesitate to include in the study patients who seem to be the best candidates for the treatment being studied. This would be the case, for example, when a patient might stand being put in a control group (waiting group or placebo group), and thus not receive the treatment. In this sort of situation there is a high probability that a number of patients will not be referred to the study by the clinicians (Candy et al. 1972).

The use of research methodologies which employ treatment sequences, such as single-case designs (Götestam, this volume), could be indicated. This, at least sometimes, permits the clinician to modify treatment strategies without eliminating the patient from the study. It is not only the general design that may affect the subject of the study; the ways in which the data are collected have to be considered too. As in any treatment evaluation we have to answer some basic questions: Who receives what, and with what result? In other words, we need a description and classification of the patient's troubles, identification of the treatment given, and evaluation of the results observed.

Identification of Depressed Patients

There are different possible attitudes to identifying a psychological illness. Those that will be discussed here are recognition of the illness, description of the psychopathology, and identification based on the opinion of the clinicians.

Recognition. To be able to recognize the illness means that – in our opinion – something must exist that has some consistency through time, and that may be recognized by a professional. This recognition would give the key to the therapeutic decisions. The implicit assumption is that there "really" is such an object that is more or less independent of the theories explaining its appearance and evolution.

As we know, this model has proved its efficacy over time – it is often called the medical model. It has shown its efficacy especially when we work on such rather concrete objects as the so-called somatic illnesses. We know now that even in this privileged field the medical model has shown its limitations, namely concerning the interaction of biological and psychological factors. This model is rather difficult to use when our objects lose their apparent stability. It seems more and more obvious that the objects are constructions, with all the concomitant advantages and disadvantages. The objects with which we are working in psychotherapy research are constructions and thus modifiable for operational purposes. The task of diagnosing the patient has caused much controversy and resulted in many publications, e.g. Akiskal (1983), Feighner et al. (1972), Frank (1969), Katz and Hirschfeld (1978), Kendell (1968), and Woodruff et al. (1974).

At least the medical model has the great advantages of simplicity and stability. It is easy to train clinicians to conform to the rules of identification, and the inter-rater agreement can be very high. However, in order to use this model we have to neglect a number of pieces of information and, worse, by the very mode of data collection we must destroy a certain amount of information, namely that connected with the therapist–patient relationship. This seems most undesirable if one wishes to study a process in which this relationship is probably determinant (Cassiers 1981).

Description. The above may at least partially explain the interest in the description of psychopathology, which attempts to make this description "objective." However, an implicit assumption here is that there exists an object which pre-exists the observer. Another assumption is that exhaustive observation will allow the observer to grasp the nature of the object. It is clear that there is no such thing as exhaustive observation; the object is always *au-delà,* it always eludes us.

The objects to be observed are chosen according to the subjective opinion of the observer or according to the points emphasized in his or her theory. In this we are far from the objectivity often claimed, for example, in support of such methods as rating scales. This said, rating scales may be useful tools at a rather gross level of description as long as we do not forget that they cannot give us more information than we have allowed them to produce. These methods can permit comparisons which could not otherwise be done.

Clinician's Opinion. Let us hope that the diagnosis has something to do with the patient, and that it does not merely reflect the theoretical doctrines of the therapist. Lest this idea appear as some sort of bad joke, I ask the reader to pause for a minute and think; some colleague will probably come to mind. I make this point to emphasize that the state of the patient (the object) as well as the attitude of the therapist (the observer) are of importance. The "attitude" of the observer is not only influenced by his or her theoretical system of reference, but also by the cultural environment, and, at least sometimes, by his or her emotional dispositions. In speaking of emotional factors I am not essentially thinking of feelings of love or hate toward the patient, but also of the emotions connected somehow with the decision-making process (Kendell 1973).

The diagnosis appears then as "something that someone tells me somewhere at some moment in time about somebody." Thus the information to be classified is what we are told by the clinician about the patient; this information concerns the patient less than it concerns the therapist's image of the patient, this image being linked to the therapeutic decision. Diagnosis per se is unusable information if we do not take into account the above-mentioned factors and if we do not try to elucidate the clinical predictions that are always present – explicit or implicit – in any decision, and especially in any indication as to treatment.

Identification of the Treatment

When we want to compare the effect of two treatments we usually have to accept the information from the therapist as to the type of treatment applied. We have to accept this information without control, because we have no means of controlling it. But we have reason to suspect that psychological treatments are distributed on a continuum. We know that our classification of treatments is arbitrary, but we should not forget that it also fluctuates. There is a great debate as to the specific or non-specific interventing factors (Frank 1971, 1974; Strupp and Hadley 1979; Derubeis et al. 1982). According to some studies the patient–therapist relation can differ more between two therapists who adhere to the same doctrine than between two therapists who claim to be of different doctrines, but who share a comparable amount of experience.

In the sixties numerous studies, for the most part content analyses, attempted to analyse the therapeutic process (e.g. Auld and Murray 1955; Dollard and Auld 1959; Gill et al. 1968; Gottschalk 1977; Marsden 1971). Interest in this sort of study seems to have almost disappeared, perhaps because the objective was too ambitious. A more modest aim would be to develop a simple but systematic typology of interaction processes. The need for this sort of tool becomes evident when we consider the empirical characterization of psychotherapy used in certain studies. It does not seem impossible to develop reliable instruments for analysing interaction (Hermann and Hovaguimian 1983). These instruments should be founded on phenomenological criteria acceptable to researchers of different doctrines, as emphasized by Gerin (1984).

In addition to an analytical approach to interactions occurring in treatment which give access to some aspect of the process, it would be of interest, and perhaps necessary, to gather hard data concerning length, frequency, rhythm and regularity of the sessions, and duration of the treatment episodes. This would allow us to define patterns of care and their typology. The temporal structure of care could then be defined (Herman and Tricot 1984) and its relation to outcome investigated.

The Results

When someone asks for aid it is probably because they need some change in life (as well in body and/or in mind) and cannot achieve it by themselves. An agreement has to be reached between patient and therapist as to the results to be achieved. This desired change is the target that we have to grasp.

As it seemed almost impossible to define such targets, researchers were led to the model of outcome studies, well illustrated by the so-called "black box" model where we simply compare two states, before treatment and after treatment. There is no need to know what happened in between. We merely have to have a sufficient number of patients, homegeneous in some regards, and describe them according to the same criteria and with the same tools. The nature of the variables and the scales of measurement usually used permit the utilization of control groups. This model, of greater or less sophistication, may give solid answers to simple questions, as illustrated by the diagnosis exercises where quite a good consensus is achieved when using a rather simple diagnosis scale (Shepherd et al. 1968; Hermann and Rossel 1979). Obviously, unless we know what we want to measure, and why, we cannot choose appropriate scales. Nevertheless, at a rather gross level one may hope that the bias in the collection of the data is negligible.

The more we refine these studies, the more we are exposed to the risk evoked by Helen Sargent (1961) of "trivial studies of correlations between isolated variables, operationally redefined beyond recognition." With this method, what we hope to gain in rigour, we often lose in meaning, in this case in clinical meaning. This was illustrated by the interviews of leading American researchers in the field by Bergin and Strupp (1970, 1972), which underlined the gap between research and practice. This gap led to the "flight from outcome into process," a phrase coined by Hoch and Zubin.

There is strong evidence that outcome studies and process studies are opposed and incompatible if done at the same time. Yet both are necessary. They pertain to different epistemological contexts, the former working on the appearances of supposed real objects, the latter on the representation of the phenomenon that we have constructed.

Process

Coming back to process studies, and it seems that they are more appropriate studies for depressive states as they are closer to clinical practice, we are confronted not only with their complexity, but also with the difficulty of proving our hypothesis in the context of justification of research. It is obvious that here the use of the usual control group is difficult, and with some methodological designs impossible (Gerin 1984).

Process studies can be done on a limited number of patients, as there are often numerous variables. However, they must not be confounded with case studies where the clinical explanation, no matter how refined and pertinent, cannot be refuted. A number of studies, especially those by Malan (1963; Malan et al. 1968, 1975), Horwitz (1974), and Brockington et al. (1982), have shown that some sort of proof may be achieved by the use of predictive models. The use of predictive models allows the introduction into the design of a number of variables, connected, for example, with the interaction between patient and therapist. In their construction they require the intervention of the theory which obviously has something to do with the decision-making process. Predictive models are fashioned according to theory and are sometimes mediated by the clinical experience of the therapist.

It is worth underlining that there are different types of prediction. The predictions we are dealing with here are conjectural (based on a model constructed according to theoretical elements) and are not merely predictions (or descriptions) based on a high correlation ratio, or even on cluster or discriminant analyse. These conjectural predictions are not necessarily ponctual (i.e., predictive of a single isolated trait), predictive trees may be constructed. The analogy with decision trees is probably not only fortuitous.

Conclusion

As we have seen, there are no specific methodological requirements in research on psychological treatments of depression. Nevertheless, the clinical particularities of depressive states and the possible severity of their evolution leads us to emphasize some design aspects, the most important of which is the need to remain close to the usual treatment procedures. The most important questions with which researchers are confronted are closely connected to clinical practice. Such questions are:

- Are certain depressive states more amenable to the psychotherapeutic approach?
- If so, what are the characteristics of depressive states most amenable to psychotherapy?
- Which forms of psychotherapy are the most useful in depressive states?
- In mixed pharmacological and psychotherapeutic treatments, what is the role of the psychotherapy or the psychological – relational dimension, and what is the role of the medication in the effects obtained?
- Is there a question of timing in the utilization of these two therapeutic approaches?
- Are there therapeutic procedures which would reduce return rates?

The studies addressing these questions are not cited here, since our purpose was to discuss the matter at a methodological level. Several references may be found in the review papers cited above.

Three of the points made above should be stressed: Diagnosis should have predictive value, in other words should be an efficient predictive tool, or it is worthless (Woodruff et al. 1974). The identification of different types of psychological treatments by criteria that do not merely reflect the theoretical representation of the observer is necessary if we want to compare the effects of different treatments and define the clinical criteria that patients have to fulfill to be eligible for a particular type of treatment. Finally, the assessment of results is the area which is most influenced by the special methodologies required by research in depressive states. As we have seen, we have to remain close to clinical practice; this leads to the choice of designs constructed on the process model, at least when we want to answer some rather finely defined questions.

Theory has its place in therapeutic decisions; it should not interfere in the description of the patient or of the treatment procedure, although these different approaches are interrelated. This raises fundamental methodological problems, especially about the reciprocal places of outcome studies and of process studies.

1. Are process studies and outcome studies compatible, or should their designs be completely different? More specifically, does an outcome study designed with the appropriate methodology (with the kind of definition of data generally used in such studies) allow us to conduct a process study?
2. What are the types of question that may be approached by these two types of study?

In other words, should we consider that population or outcome studies developed according to models used in the biological sciences are the only ones able to give unambiguous answers? And that process studies are worth using merely as pilot studies? Or should we think that predictive process studies are the only ones that give access to the complexity of what occurs between patient and therapist in the therapeutic relationship? This is only acceptable if we think that predictive process studies are studies in which theory is the matrix upon which the clinical models are built, the clinical models in turn directing clinical decision making. This would mean that outcome studies should be reserved for rather gross questions in which the bias in collection of standardized data on a number of people may be considered as negligible.

Research studies in the field of the psychological treatment of depressive states will probably increase during the years to come, not only because of the frequency of depressive states, and the important clinical problems raised by their treatment, but also because of the importance and the acuteness of the methodological problems that they raise.

References

Akiskal HS (1983) Dysthymic disorders: psychopathology of proposed chronic depressive subtypes. Am J Psychiatry 140:11–19

Akiskal HS, McKinney WT (1975) Overview of recent research in depression. Arch Gen Psychiatry 32:285–305

Ariety S, Bemporad J (1980) Severe and mild depression. The psychotherapeutic approach. Tavistock, London

Auld F, Murray EJ (1955) Content-analysis studies of psychotherapy. Psychol Bull 52:377–395

Becker J, Schuckit MA (1978) The comparative efficacy of cognitive therapy and pharmacotherapy in the treatment of depressions. Cog Ther Res 2:193–197

Bergin AE, Strupp HH (1970) New directions in psychotherapy research. J Abnorm Psychol 76:13–26

Bergin AE, Strupp HH (1972) Changing frontiers in the science of psychotherapy. Aldine Press, Chicago

Brockington IF, Helzer JE, Hillier VP, Francis AF (1982) Definitions of depression: Concordance and prediction of outcome. Am J Psychiatry 139:1022–1027

Candy J, Balfour FHG, Cawley RH, Hildebrand HP, Malan DH, Marks IM, Wilson J (1972) A feasibility study of a controlled trial of formal psychotherapy. Psychol Med 2:345–362

Cassiers L (1981) La dépression. Point de vue psychothérapeutique. Arch Belg Med Soc 39:87–95

Cronholm B, Daly RJ (1983) Evaluation of psychiatric treatment. In: Helgason T (ed) Methodology in evaluation of psychiatric treatment. Cambridge University Press, Cambridge

Derubeis RS, Hollon SD, Evans MD, Bemis KM (1982) Can psychotherapies for depression be discriminated? A systematic investigation of cognitive therapy and interpersonal therapy. J Consult Clin Psychol 50:744–756

Dollard J, Auld F (1959) Previous studies bearing on content analysis of psychotherapy. In: Scoring human motives: a manual. Yale University Press, New Haven

Feighner JP, Robins E, Guze SB, Woodruff RA, Winokur G, Munoz R (1972) Diagnostic criteria for use in psychiatric research. Arch Gen Psychiat 26:57–63

Frank GH (1969) Psychiatric diagnosis: A review of research. J Gen Psychol 81:157–176

Frank JD (1971) Therapeutic factors in psychotherapy. Am J Psychother 25:350–361

Frank JD (1974) Therapeutic components of psychotherapy. J Nerv Ment Dis 159:325–342

Gerin P (1984) L'évaluation des psychothérapies. PUF, Paris

Gill MM, Simon J, Fink G, Endicott NA, Paul IH (1968) Studies in audio-recorded psychoanalysis. J Am Psychoanal Assoc 16:230–244

Gomes-Schwartz B (1978) Effective ingredients in psychotherapy: prediction of outcome from process variables. J Consult Clin Psychol 46:1023–1035

Gottschalk LA (1977) Recent advances in the content analysis of speech and the application of this measurement approach to psychosomatic research. Psychother Psychosom 28:73–82

Haynal A (1983) La psychothérapie de la dépression. Med Psychosom 4:206–211

Hermann P (1983) Idéologies et modèles en psychothérapie. Psychothérapies 4:215–228

Hermann P (1984) La prise de décision Médicale. Psychol Méd 16:599–604

Hermann P, Hovaguimian T (1983) Une méthode d'évaluation des interventions du thérapeute dans le cadre d'entretiens à visée psychothérapique. Ann Méd Psychol 141:601–605

Hermann P, Rossel Y (1979) Les exercices diagnostiques. Méd Hygiène 37:3031–3041

Hermann P, Tricot L (1984) Une méthode d'analyse de la structure temporelle des traitements. WHO

Holton G (1973) Thematic origin of scientific thought. Harvard University Press, Cambridge

Holton G (1978) The scientific imagination: case studies. Cambridge University Press, Cambridge

Horwitz L (1974) Clinical predictions in psychotherapy. Aronson, New York

Katz MM, Hirschfeld MA (1978) Phenomenology and classification of depression. In: Lipton MA, Dimascio A, Killam KF (eds) Psycho-pharmacology: a generation of progress. Rosen, New York

Keithly LJ, Samples SJ, Strupp HH (1980) Patient motivation as a predictor of process and outcome in psychotherapy. Psychother Psychosom 33:87–97

Keller MB, Klerman GL, Lavori PW, Fawcett JA, Coryell W, Endicott J (1982) Treatment received by depressed patients. Jama 248:1848–1855

Kendell RE (1968) The classification of depressive illnesses. Oxford University Press, Oxford

Kendell RE (1973) Psychiatric diagnoses: A study of how they are made. Br J Psychiatry 122:437–445

Klerman GL et al. (1974) Treatment of depression by drugs and psychotherapy. Am J Psychiatry 131:186–191

Lambert MJ (1979) The effects of psychotherapy. Churchill Livingstone, Edinburgh

Malan DH (1963) A study of brief psychotherapy. Thomas, London

Malan DH, Bacal HA, Heath ES, Balfour FHG (1968) A study of psychodynamic changes in untreated neurotic patients – I. Br J Psychiatry 114:525–551

Malan DH, Heath ES, Bacal HA, Balfour FHG (1975) Psychodynamic changes in untreated neurotic patients – II. Arch Gen Psychiatry 32:110–126

Marsden G (1971) Content-analysis studies of psychotherapy: 1954 through 1968. In: Bergin AE, Garfield SL (eds) Handbook of psychotherapy and behavior change. Wiley, New York

Rehm LP, Kornblith SJ (1979) Behavior therapy for depression. A review of recent development. Prog Behav Modification 7:277–318

Reichenbach H (1938) Experience and prediction. University of Chicago Press, Chicago

Sargent HD (1961) Intrapsychic change: methodological Problems in psychotherapy research. Psychiatry 24:93–108

Sartorius N (1975) Epidemiology of depression. WHO Chron 29:423–427

Schmale AH (1958) Relationship of separation and depression to disease. Psychosom Med 20:259–277

Schmale AH, Iker HP (1965) The affect of hopelessness and the development of cancer. Psychosom Med 28:714–721

Schmale AH, Iker HP (1971) Hopelessness as a predictor of cervical cancer. Soc Sci Med 5:95–100

Schneider P-B (1978) Psychothérapie de la dépression. Rev Méd Suisse Romande 98:489–498

Seligman MEP, Klein DC, Miller WR (1976) Depression. In: Leitenberg H (ed) Handbook of behaviour modification and behaviour therapy. Munksgaard, Copenhagen

Shepherd M, Brooke EM, Cooper JE, Lin T (1968) An experimental approach to psychiatric diagnosis. Acta Psychiatr Scand 44 (suppl 201): 1–89

Strupp HH, Hadley SW (1979) Specific vs non specific factors in Psychotherapy: A controlled study of outcome. Arch Gen Psychiatry 6:1125–1136

Taylor FG, Marshall WL (1977) Experimental analysis of a cognitive-behavioral therapy for depression. Cog Ther Res 1:59–72

Weissmann MM (1979) The psychological treatment of depression. Arch Gen Psychiatry 36:1261–1269

Whitehead A (1979) Psychological treatment of depression: a review. Behav Res Ther 17:495–509

Woodruff RA, Goodwing DW, Guze SB (1974) Psychiatric diagnosis. Oxford University Press, Oxford

Family Therapy of Alcoholism: An Evaluation of Its Efficiency as a Predetoxification Move

J. P. Roussaux[1]

Introduction

The case material in this study comes from two institutions located in Brussels (Belgium), the Institut Neurologique Belge (INB) and the Adult Guidance Center (AGC). Both are parts of the Department of Psychiatry in the Catholic University of Louvain. For 4 years we have been working regularly with alcoholics and their families. Our work is based on the following hypotheses:

a) Alcohol is an organizing factor in the functioning of an "alcoholic family" (Steinglass 1980)
b) The individual who drinks helps to organize around him- or herself a series of rituals that result in behaviours predictable by the family, that in some way resolve other difficulties that exist and that "need" not be dealt with immediately (Davis et al. 1974)
c) Therapy directed toward immediate detoxification puts the therapist into a symmetrical relationship with the alcohol abuser and his or her family; it creates either a total separation or an escalation in the abuse (Borwick 1982)

It is possible to divide the therapeutic process into three parts: (1) negotiation before and during detoxification, which creates a stimulating support for the family; (2) detoxification in a specialized clinic for 2 weeks, during which period at least one meeting with the family is scheduled; (3) therapy to support change in the family after the hospitalization. In this study, we will try to establish how the use of family therapy in the predetoxification stage can increase significantly not only the completion of the detoxification phase, but also the acceptance by the family and the "dry" alcoholic patient of a follow-through therapy. As an ultimate consequence, this manoeuvre increases the abstinence rate. The psychodynamic reasons for such effects will not be developed or discussed in this paper.

Material and Method

The 40 patients in the study were all white men and women aged between 27 and 65 years. They came from the same area (south of Brussels) and the same

[1] Université Catholique de Louvain, Service de Psychiatrie, 30 Clos Chapelle-aux-Champs, Bte 3049, B-1200 Bruxelles

Psychological Treatment of Mental Illness
Edited by R. J. Daly and E. A. Sand

social class (lower middle). To enter the study, they had to have been married or living with the same partner for at least 3 years. All patients had volunteered for detoxification, and all had an alcohol dependence (D. S. M. III:303–91) and a previous history of alcohol withdrawal symptoms (D. S. M. III:291–80). None was psychotic and none had irreversible liver or brain disease.

The initial sample of 40 patients was divided into two groups of 20 patients each, according to the first treatment received. The first group consisted of patients and their families whose demands for detoxification were not satisfied at once, but only after several family therapy sessions (from 3 to 8). These patients used to come directly to the AGC, where the predetoxification family sessions always took place. The patient was then referred to the detoxification ward in the INB. The second group consisted of patients who had been immediately admitted to the detoxification ward (INB) without any systematic family interview. They were seen for the first time at the INB. For both groups, the detoxification was always conducted at the INB using the classical medical method (sedation, hydration, B vitamins). At entry each patient was asked to agree to and sign a written contract, the conditions of which included staying for a minimum of 14 days, of which the first 7 days were to be spent in isolation from the outside world and particularly from the family. The contract was considered broken in cases of violence, drinking or unauthorized departure from the ward.

The family therapy sessions lasted 1 hour. They were directed by one therapist for couples and by two therapists for families. Children over 12 years were asked to at least one session. For both groups a family meeting was arranged during the hospitalization. For patients of the second group this constituted the first family therapy session. All patients were encouraged during the hospitalization to attend at least at one meeting of Alcoholics Anonymous (A. A.), held inside the clinic.

The measure of individual evolution chosen was total abstinence until the sixth month after hospital release (after a longer period this measure of amelioration would probably be less valid; Miller 1983). The information was obtained from both the patient and family. The measure chosen for the rest of the family, mainly the spouse, was their own rating of their state after 6 months. They were asked to answer the question "Did the whole process have a positive effect (+), negative effect (−), or no effect (0) on your own situation?"

Results and Comments

The results for individual patients are given in Tables 1 and 2. The first important difference between the groups concerns fulfilment of the detoxification contract. Patients who had family interviews before admission did better in the detoxification itself; they all fulfilled their contract (100%) in comparison with only 65% of the second group.

Table 1. Treatment and results for the group receiving family therapy before detoxification (group 1)

Case no.	Sex	Age	No. of family therapy sessions before detoxification	Fulfilment of contract	No. of family therapy sessions after detoxification	Regular attendance of A.A.	Abstinence	Family self-evaluation
1	M	43	4	+	10	–	+	+
2	M	62	3	+	12	+	+	+
3	M	31	3	+	6	–	+	+
4	M	32	8	+	8	+	+	+
5	M	51	3	+	7	–	+	+
6	M	54	4	+	1	+	+	+
7	F	34	5	+	1	–	–	–
8	M	42	4	+	5	–	+	+
9	M	54	5	+	1	–	–	0
10	M	57	3	+	0	–	–	0
11	M	53	3	+	1	+	+	+
12	M	31	3	+	7	–	+	+
13	M	52	3	+	0	–	–	0
14	M	38	4	+	5	–	+	+
15	M	33	5	+	11	–	+	+
16	F	41	3	+	8	–	–	+
17	M	45	3	+	8	–	+	+
18	F	37	4	+	0	–	–	–
19	M	41	4	+	1	–	–	–
20	F	43	3	+	11	+	+	+

It is known that length of time spent in treatment is a major predictor of treatment outcome. Families and patients in the first group were more likely to continue the family therapy after detoxification was completed. The mean number of therapy sessions attended over 6 months by patients in group 1 was 5.15, compared with 1.3 sessions for patients in group 2. It is also important to note that more patients in the first group regularly visited an A. A. group (25% versus 20%).

The most important result is that the group 1 patients showed a much better abstinence rate after 6 months than the group 2 patients (65% versus 30%). A less striking but nevertheless significant result is the difference in family satisfaction: 70% satisfaction in group 1 compared with 40% in group 2.

Conclusions

This study gives a quantitative basis to the increasingly common clinical conviction that family therapy is an effective method of treatment in the general

Table 2. Treatment and results for the group receiving no family therapy before detoxification (group 2)

Case no.	Sex	Age	No. of family therapy sessions before detoxification	Fulfilment of contract	No. of family therapy sessions after detoxification	Regular attendance of A.A.	Abstinence	Family self-evaluation
1	M	31	0	+	0	–	–	0
2	M	28	0	–	0	–	–	0
3	M	52	0	+	0	–	+	+
4	M	34	0	+	6	–	+	+
5	M	43	0	+	0	+	–	0
6	M	41	0	–	4	–	–	+
7	M	51	0	–	2	–	–	0
8	M	43	0	–	8	–	+	+
9	M	46	0	+	1	–	–	0
10	M	27	0	–	1	–	–	–
11	M	52	0	+	2	+	+	+
12	M	41	0	+	0	–	–	0
13	M	38	0	+	3	–	–	+
14	M	46	0	–	0	–	–	–
15	M	28	0	+	6	–	–	–
16	F	42	0	+	7	+	+	+
17	M	41	0	+	0	+	–	0
18	F	38	0	+	4	–	–	0
19	M	65	0	+	2	–	+	+
20	M	31	0	–	0	–	–	–

field of addiction (Roussaux 1982; Stanton and Todd 1982) and particularly for alcoholism (Cassiers 1983). Our main point is that family therapy is more effective if it is started before the detoxification phase of the therapeutic process. As a consequence, hospitalization for detoxification should not remain the culminating point of the treatment, but should be regarded only as a technical procedure necessary to achieve certain issues that are correct for the individual and for the family.

References

Borwick B (1982) Consultations préliminaires dans le traitement de l'alcoolique. Thér Fam 3:201–213

Cassiers L (1983) Fonction familiale de l'alcoolisme. Thér Fam 3:291– 305

Davis DI et al. (1974) The adaptive consequences of drinking. Psychiatry 37:209–216

Miller WR (1983) Controlled drinking: history and a critical review. J Stud Alcohol 44

Roussaux JP (1982) Familles d'héroïnomanes en thérapie. Thér Fam 3:257–269

Stanton MD, Todd TC (1982) The family therapy of drug abuse and addiction. Guilford, New York

Steinglass P (1980) A life history model of the alcoholic family. Fam Process 19:211–226

Preliminary Studies of an Evaluation Research of Psychotherapies*

J. BOVET[1]

At the University Psychiatric Policlinic of Lausanne we intend to study prospectively the outcomes of psychotherapies done there. The Policlinic is an exclusively outpatient public service, open to every psychiatric patient whose troubles do not necessitate hospitalization. Such patients may be psychotic, alcoholic, neurotic, etc. The psychotherapies are reserved for patients with neurotic or allied troubles. They are of Freudian inspiration, but may assume different forms: brief or without time limit, individual or group, supportive or "uncovering", etc.

As yet, we have not started the outcome study itself, having only collected the necessary data from about 80 patients, without analyzing them. However, we have set up the method, i.e. the principles and the instruments by which we intend to conduct our research.

Concerning the principles, we aim for as little interference as possible between the research and ordinary therapeutic practice. We have also chosen to collect our information at the beginning and at the end of treatment and, whenever we are able, at some follow-up points (one, two or more years after the end of treatment).

As for the instruments we are using, there are two, and both are applied only to the patients (the therapist takes no part in the study). These instruments are a version of the Semantic Differential test of Osgood, and a clinical "questionnaire", derived from those of Sifneos, to be answered by the patient.

The Semantic Differential, which is a sort of projective test with a verbal content, aims to determine the connotative (or affective) meaning of words, or of the underlying concepts. Each concept chosen is evaluated on a series of adjectival scales (we have 30); the information on the scales can be reduced by factor analysis. We have found three main factors, very similar to the three classical ones of Osgood, and have labelled them evaluation, potency and activity. This three-factor structure lends itself to quite informative graphic representation. We chose to submit 11 words for evaluation: *mother, father, myself, woman, man, child, future, dream, sex, guilty,* and *death.*

* Research supported by the Fonds national suisse de la recherche scientifique (No. 3.921-080).

[1] Centre de Recherche de l'Institut Universitaire d'Hygiène Mentale, Rue César Roux 29, CH-1005 Lausanne.

Psychological Treatment of Mental Illness
Edited by R. J. Daly and E. A. Sand

There are many advantages to the Semantic Differential. As it is not affected by any learning process, it can be repeated at brief or long intervals. It can be applied to anybody, regardless of whether they are a patient or not, psychotic or neurotic, with or without treatment, etc.; hence it is possible for the results to be placed in very general frames of reference. The filling out of the scales by the subjects is very simple. The processing of the raw data may be more or less sophisticated, but in any event, it is of a "hard" type, entirely communicable and reproducible. The disadvantages of the Semantic Differential are those of any projective (or disguised) technique, and indeed of any test (even of intelligence), and mainly concern the difficulty of linking the results to the patient's reality, in other words of giving the results a valuable clinical meaning.

The clinical questionnaire consists of 25–30 questions about the patient's complaints, relationships (past and present), faculties of insight, motivation to change and appreciation of treatment after it is completed. Unlike Sifneos, who asked these questions of objective raters, we ask the patients themselves, requesting written answers. It is worth remarking that this seldom provokes any difficulty. The validity of these questionnaires (i.e. their adequacy to obtain data relevant to the clinic) is, by their very nature, much more obvious than that of the Semantic Differential. However, they do have some disadvantages. They can only be applied to patients following a psychotherapy, thus restricting the possibilities for large frames of reference. Their analysis is complex and partly of a "soft" type. Since the questions are open, the answers can show large variations of length, style and content; in order to get valid comparisons, we use a form of content analysis, according to a scheme proposed long ago by Lasswell, a psychoanalyst.

As yet, we have not started to apply our instruments to the prospective study of a sample of patients from the beginning to the end of their psychotherapy. However, we have done many preliminary studies and trials on other samples, and here I will point out briefly some results using the Semantic Differential.

Among the indications of the internal validity of the Semantic Differential, the matching of tests to retests is worth mentioning. If one has, say, 100 tests of 100 subjects in a particular order and 100 retests of the same subjects (taken many weeks or months after the first tests) in a different order, random relative to the first, one can match the test and retest of each individual at a very high rate (between 75% and 90%), either intuitively by looking at graphic representations of the semantic configurations, or by using a computer program. Such a finding shows that the semantic configuration reflects some traits identifying the individuals.

If we compare statistically samples of "normal", neurotic and schizophrenic subjects, we find some interesting differences. On the first axis (evaluation, "good – bad"), the mean evaluation of neurotics is more negative ("pessimistic") for the five words that usually refer to personal experience (*mother, father, myself, future* and *dream*) whereas their evaluation of the words which are usually felt on a more impersonal, cultural register (*woman, man, child* and *death*) is much more like that of normal subjects. On the second axis (potency) we find that the mean relative evaluation of the words *myself* and *guilty* is inverted in neurotic patients (*guilty*, positive ["strong"]; *myself*, negative ["weak"]; the evaluation is opposite in normal and schizophrenic subjects). In addition, the variance of the samples of patients – mainly neurotics – is often larger than that of normal people, reflecting, it may be supposed, the variety of affective and relational problems underlying their psychopathology.

The evolution over time, estimated by test–retest, is often significantly less in a sample of normal people (over a time interval of 9–16 months) than in a sample of neurotics following a psychotherapy (over a time interval of 5–11 months during the course of a therapy). We cannot yet say whether the treatment plays some role in this greater change, or whether neurotics are more prone to change with or without treatment.

Psychotherapy Research on Schizophrenia

P. TIENARI[1]

Introduction

As a general definition, psychotherapy should be seen as a treatment in which the relationship between patient and therapist provides a context for understanding of psychological components of illness and the psychosocial matrix of its development. While there are major cognitive or intellectual components in developing self-understanding, most forms of psychotherapy presume that the emotional components of the therapeutic relationship are indispensable in accumulating information and assimilating insight (Heinrichs and Carpenter 1981). There are several reasons to demand reconsideration of the role of psychotherapy in the treatment of schizophrenia. Among the possible contributing factors are the growing interest in biological models of aetiology, the success of antipsychotic drugs, the increased emphasis on rigorous empirical research methods, and a public policy that spreads fixed mental health resources across the largest possible number of patients.

Theories of the Aetiology of Schizophrenia

Biological and genetic factors are important parts of the puzzle of schizophrenic aetiology. In the ongoing nurture-nature debate, evidence for these factors has frequently been linked with the assumption that aetiology should define treatment (Soskis 1972). There has been a growing realization that aetiology itself is complex and must be conceptualized in terms of interactions of multiple factors, some which are genetic and biological and others which are psychological and environmental in nature (Strauss and Carpenter 1981; Tienari et al. 1985a, b). The question of the validity of psychodynamic views of the pathogenesis of schizophrenia is quite different from the issue of effectiveness of psychodynamic psychotherapy. Furthermore, confirmation of biological factors in the aetiology of schizophrenia undermines psychogenic theory and psychotherapy practice only to the extent that psychological and sociological factors are hypothesized as incompatible with biological aetiology. The biopsychosocial medical model provides a framework for integrating

[1] Department of Psychiatry, University of Oulu, SF-90210 Oulu 21, Finland

Psychological Treatment of Mental Illness
Edited by R. J. Daly and E. A. Sand

these seemingly diverse attributes in conceptualizing schizophrenia (Carpenter et al. 1983; Carpenter 1984).

Family therapy has been useful in the treatment of schizophrenia (Falloon 1982; Stierlin et al. 1983). However, as several reviews have noted, the vast majority of empirical attempts to differentiate the families of schizophrenics from other families have been either unsuccessful or inconsistent. The primary exception, communication deviance, is an intriquing variable that lends itself to several interpretations, including a genetic one (Wynne et al. 1977; Liem 1980).

While the question of aetiology has played an important role in theoretical discussions of schizophrenia, the single factor having the most profound impact on practice has been the development of antipsychotic drugs. Not every schizophrenic patient responds to or requires antipsychotic drugs, but the majority benefit from them. Antipsychotic drugs have proved to be powerful in reducing and preventing psychotic symptoms, but they have not been clearly efficacious in dealing with the interpersonal and occupational limitations of patients or with deficit symptoms.

The setting for treatment has changed profoundly. Brief hospitalizations have replaced long-term hospital-based care. The patient returns to the community, and, if treatment is continued, it is most often in a public clinic in which therapeutic resources are limited. This contrasts sharply with the traditional notion of psychotherapeutic work with the schizophrenic patient. Such work has usually implied intensive involvement between patient and therapist over many years. Extended periods of regression would require considerable management, often in the hospital setting. Similarly, the hospital setting would guarantee that the therapist had continued access to the patient, even when the patient was hostile and rejecting. Quite apart from the question of validity of traditional models of psychotherapy, the manner in which they have usually been practised is no longer directly applicable to the typical schizophrenic patient. Thus, it has become necessary to demonstrate that the psychotherapeutic strategies can be effectively modified to deal with the current treatment setting. Psychotherapy compares poorly with antipsychotic drugs in rapid reduction of psychotic symptoms, but the effects of each treatment on social functioning and deficit symptoms are relatively unexplored. The question then becomes, how much additional benefit can be obtained from psychotherapy in resolving residual symptoms of the illness. Although such symptoms may often significantly impair the schizophrenic's functioning, attempting psychotherapy is no longer the obvious solution, given its cost and the uncertainty of its results. The emergence of antipsychotic drugs requires a new framework for thinking about psychotherapy. Psychotherapeutic strategies now have a role in a more comprehensive treatment strategy, and they focus on those objectives to which psychotherapy can make unique contributions. Treatment is now made in a context that permits a rapid return to some level of independent functioning and must have a reasonable likelihood of success at an acceptable cost (Heinrichs and Carpenter 1982).

Review of Psychotherapy Research

Two early controlled psychotherapy studies have been published (Bookhammer 1966; Fairweather et al. 1960). These were pioneer works, but design does not permit evaluation of the efficacy of psychotherapy on schizophrenia. Rogers et al. (1967) studied 32 hospitalized schizophrenics. Patients were randomly assigned to psychotherapy or no psychotherapy conditions and an attempt was made to minimize the use of medication in those receiving psychotherapy. There was no significant difference between client-centred therapy patients and controls. Those who received psychotherapy showed only very modest advantages over those who did not after 18 months, i.e. they had less residivism in the year following discharge.

Grinspoon et al. (1972) published a study where chronic patients were treated twice weekly by experienced psychotherapists over a 2-year period. Half of these patients received pharmacotherapy in addition to psychotherapy, and half received psychotherapy alone. These 20 experimental subjects were selected from among 41 single males who had been hospitalized. Random design was attempted, but "experimental" patients who refused, or whose families refused, to change hospitals were reassigned to the control group. The control group remained in the state hospital on phenothiazines. The experimental patients were transferred to a new and unfamiliar setting, the Massachusetts Mental Health Center. The group receiving psychotherapy alone did significantly worse than the group who also received drugs and showed no advantages when compared with a similar group of patients who had chosen to remain in a custodial setting. Conclusions from this study were limited because of the chronic nature of the illness and the absence of a randomly assigned comparison.

Karon and VandenBos (1981) randomly assigned 36 hospitalized schizophrenics to psychotherapy alone, psychotherapy plus drugs or drugs alone. The psychotherapy-without-medication group received an active psychoanalytic psychotherapy, the group receiving both therapy and drugs was given "ego-analytic" psychotherapy, and the third group was hospitalized in a public institution in which phenothiazines were used as a primary treatment. The two psychotherapy groups had significantly shorter hospital stays and performed significantly better on clinical status interviews, as well as on a number of performance tests, when compared with the group treated in the maintainance milieu programme. However, it was not possible to determine whether these advantages were due to the psychotherapy, to uncontrolled variations in medication, or to the radically different hospital programme in which the comparison group was treated.

May (1968) published a well-known controlled study of five methods of treating schizophrenic patients. These treatment methods were psychotherapy without medication, psychotherapy with medication, medication alone, electroconvulsive therapy (ECT) and milieu therapy. Treatment was administered by psychiatric residents or psychiatrists without extensive experience. To control the personality factors, each psychiatrist practised each of the five methods. Patients were reported to be assigned randomly to the five treatments and those treated were first-admission, clearly schizophrenic patients, between the ages of 16 and 45, who were in the "middle third of severity." The therapy was primarily ego-supportive in nature with an emphasis on defining reality. The patients were assessed on a wide range of outcome variables. Patients were followed-up for up to 5 years. Antipsychotic drugs proved significantly superior to psychotherapy (Heinrichs and Carpenter 1981):

> This work is impressive evidence that psychotherapy administered in the hospital by inexperienced therapists to midprognostic-range schizophrenic (not selected for psychotherapy suitability) is not effective. The generalizability of this work has been challenged in the belief that a more selected group of patients or more experienced therapists would have made a difference. Nevertheless, this investigation was a telling assessment of what was then the most common psychotherapeutic experience available to the hospitalized schizophrenic patients.

The percentages of successes in each treatment group were as follows: drugs alone 96%, psychotherapy plus drug 95%, ECT 79%, psychotherapy 65% and milieu 58% (May et al. 1976a). Patients who had been originally treated in hospital with psychotherapy alone stayed longer in hospital over the follow-up period of 2–5 years than those who had received ECT, drug alone or drug plus psychotherapy (May et al. 1976b). A 3- to 5-year follow-up examined their course after release from the hospital (May et al. 1981). The drug-alone and ECT groups tended to have the best outcome and the psychotherapy-alone group the worst.

Stanton et al. (1984) and Gunderson et al. (1984) described a 2-year, multihospital study on the effects of psychotherapy for non-chronic schizophrenic patients. The design and methods were selected to evaluate the relative benefits of exploratory insight-oriented (EIO) psychotherapy and reality-adaptive supportive (RAS) psychotherapy, when both are provided by experienced therapists against the backdrop of good hospital and psychopharmacological management. Similarities and differences between the two therapies and therapists were clearly outlined. Of the 186 patients who were suitable, 164 consented to participate and were randomly assigned to treatment. Of the 164 patients who entered the study, 69 (42%) dropped out before qualifying as study patients, i.e. before completing a minimum of 6 months in their assigned treatment modality. These 69 who had dropped out of psychotherapy were studied with regard to both their reasons for dropping out and their subsequent clinical course assessed by means of a retrospective, semistructured interview (Katz et al. 1984). As a group, they received an unexpectedly substantial amount of subsequent psychiatric treatment, and after 2 years did not generally differ from those remaining in psychotherapy on measures of social and occupational functioning.

The final sample consisted of those 95 patients (43 EIO and 52 RAS) who remained in their assigned treatment condition for at least 6 months. Analyses of 2-year outcomes revealed a complex interaction between the type of psychotherapy provided and the domain of psychopathology affected. RAS psychotherapy exerted clear preferential effects in the areas of recidivism and role performance. The EIO psychotherapy exerted some preferential effects in the areas of ego functioning and cognition.

Hogarty et al. (1974) examined the role of individual social case work and vocational counselling, termed "major role therapy," in the aftercare of schizophrenic patients. After randomly assigning 374 newly discharged schizophrenics to chlorpromazine or placebo aftercare, each group was further randomly assigned to either "no psychological treatment" or "major role therapy" (MRT). Patients were treated for 2 years or until relapse. At 18 and 24 months, a significant interaction appeared between the effects of MRT and drugs, and measures of symptoms, social and occupational adjustment, and overall functioning among the subgroup of patients completing the study without relapse. For medicated patients, MRT improved functioning, especially in interpersonal relations and overall functioning. Unmedicated patients, however, did better without MRT. MRT also affected time to relapse in different ways; patients with no severe symptoms benefited from MRT, while in patients with greater symptom severity MRT, surprisingly, hastened relapse (Goldberg et al. 1977).

Suggestions for Future Studies

Selection of Subjects Appropriate to Treatment. The patients chosen should be acceptable candidates for the treatment in question. The schizophrenic disorders are very heterogeneous, and it is unlikely that any treatment would help all patients.

In the Boston psychotherapy study (Stanton et al. 1984) the seletion of a patient sample was intended to identify a mid-range prognostic group of clearly schizophrenic patients who were neither too chronic to be expected to respond to treatment nor so acute as to improve independently of the given treatment. The criteria used were as follows: The patient should (1) have been clinically diagnosed schizophrenic or probable schizophrenic by the admitting hospital psychiatrist; (2) be between the ages of 18 and 35; (3) have an IQ within the normal range (>90), show no evidence of organicity, drug or alcohol abuse and have no grossly handicapping physical illness; (4) not have received 20 or more ECT treatments in the past; (5) not be actively involved in ongoing psychotherapy or have had more than 2 years of once-weekly psychotherapy or its equivalent; (6) not have had more than 6 months of continuous hospitalization prior to the index admission; (7) have been able to function non-psychotically outside hospital without neuroleptics for at least 4 consecutive months out of the preceding 2 years; (8) show no remission of psychotic symptoms within 3 days of admission; (9) receive a second diagnosis of schizophrenia or probable schizophrenia from a research psychiatrist on the basis of standardized interview (psychiatric status schedule); (10) receive a third diagnosis of schizophrenia or probable schizophrenia by fulfilling five or more of the World Health Organization's Diagnostic Criteria for Schizophrenia (DCS).

Selection of Subjects in Appropriate Phase of Illness. Since schizophrenic illness varies over time, the selection of patients in the appropriate phase of illness is crucial for testing the efficacy of any treatment. The treatment of schizophrenia should be planned according to the problems of the particular patient. In most earlier studies, the same treatment and the same scheme were used on patients representing different phases of illness (acute, relapse, chronic, florid psychosis or negative symptoms). The critical area today is outpatient therapy.

Provision of Sufficient Levels and Duration of Treatment. Many forms of psychotherapy require a long time, with most benefits being realized late in treatment. Furthermore, individuals respond at remarkably different rates. Studies are strengthened when the psychotherapy itself is highly specified, administered by experienced therapists and of a duration and intensity likely to maximize the therapeutic change.

The advantages of psychotherapy become evident after patients have been seen for a year and a half or more. It should be provided within a supportive psychosocial context, and involve at least twice-weekly and generally more frequent meetings. Psychoanalytically oriented explorations require close supervision or an experienced, personally analysed therapist (Gunderson and Carroll 1983).

Heinrichs and Carpenter (1981) pointed out that long duration of treatment may be necessary to demonstrate benefits from some interpersonal treatments, and beneficial effects of psychological therapy may only be apparent in patients receiving medication. False negatives may be obtained in studies of too brief duration or where psychotherapy is not evaluated in combination with drug treatment. This has also been demonstrated by Goldstein et al. (1981) for a combination of drug and family therapy. They showed that 6 weeks of combined drug and crisis family therapy completely prevented rehospitalization and reduced symptoms over a 6-month period. Benefits of the brief treatments were still apparent 3–6 years later.

Establishment of Sufficient Outcome Measures. It is important to consider various domains of outcome independently when assessing effects of treatment. Only by assessing a spectrum of outcome areas can an investigator ensure that an important benefit is not being missed and determine in which areas the treatment has no effect or may, in fact, be harmful. Outcome assessment in schizophrenia research has tended to emphasize psychotic symptoms and to neglect deficit symptoms and the interpersonal and intrapsychic consequences of illness (Heinrichs and Carpenter 1982).

In the Boston psychotherapy study (Stanton et al. 1984) the authors wanted to measure the outcome of psychotherapy along a number of dimensions that had shown promise in previous studies of schizophrenia and to use a host of other measures that would capture conceptually the areas of growth and change. They wanted to pay special attention not only to the outward behavioural signs of change, but also to the kinds of intrapsychic change assumed to be more specific to the dynamically oriented therapy. In addition, an effort was made to gather data from variety of sources, including patients, therapists, significant others, ward staff, blind evaluaters and project staff. Finally, attention was given to obtaining outcome measures repeatedly and at regular intervals so that variations in the nature of changes occurring in the

EIO and RAS conditions over time could be examined. Similar considerations covered the selection and timing of process measures. The final group of measures important to their study was those antecedent characteristics of the studied patients and therapists that might be expected to affect process and outcome directly, as well as affecting outcome indirectly through their mediating effect on process.

Description of the Psychotherapies and Therapists. Schizophrenics generally have difficulty forming and sustaining relationships with others. It is possible that engaging the patient into a stable, predictable and unthreatening therapeutic relationship can be valuable in the light of the social withdrawal and avoidance that tends to characterize the illness. It remains to be demonstrated that what the therapist does has an impact over and above the effects of a supportive relationship. Many experienced therapists believe that whatever the contribution of non-specific factors common to any therapeutic relationship, these alone are insufficient to effect deep and lasting change. They contend that while warmth and acceptance may be necessary for establishing therapeutic atmosphere, specific approaches based on theories of aetiology and treatment have a greater effect. Both the theoretical approach and the personality of the therapist may well influence the outcome of treatment. Crucial factors such as patient motivation, patient–therapist matching and a strong belief shared by patient and therapist that the psychotherapy being done is the most desirable treatment option, are obvious problems affected by research design. Psychotherapy and therapists can not be standardized and monitored in detail. The efficacy of psychotherapy may be minimally dependent on the precise mode of treatment and maximally dependent on innate qualities of the therapists (Heinrichs and Carpenter 1981).

In the Boston psychotherapy study the psychotherapies were defined as follows (Stanton et al. 1984). Reality-adaptive supportive psychotherapy (RAS) was generally concerned with problems in the current living situation of the patients, there was little attempt to explore the past and seek correlates between past experience and the present, its focus was upon the patients' behaviour rather than the potential covered meaning behind the behaviour, and a major aspect was its reality supporting. Expressive insight-oriented psychotherapy (EIO) supported and utilized the schizophrenic patients' available ego functions, the purpose being the detailed exploration of the patients' inner experience and relations with others. Its aim was to increase insight, i.e. understanding of aspects of mental activity which contributed to illness and its continuation. Although linked to psychoanalytic theories of therapy and psychopathology, it was by no means psychoanalysis. EIO therapy was intended to be conducted three or more times per week.

Earlier studies have not analysed in detail who the therapists were and what they believed. Developing valid, reliable instruments to describe the therapist's theoretical model of treatment and to isolate important personality variables would help the researcher know more about the nature of the treatment administered and the dimensions that influence outcome. In the Boston psychotherapy study (Frosch et al. 1983) each therapist was asked to rate himself on a 7-point scale with points 1, 4 and 7 anchored. Points 1 and 7 represented extreme points of view. In general, low ratings indicated adherence to a strict psychoanalytic approach, while high ratings indicated a supportive maintainance approach. This method of characterizing the therapists' theoretical beliefs was developed by conducting semistructured interviews with therapists who were not participating in the study.

The EIO therapists believed in the importance of developmental factors in treatment and aetiology, in the alterability of the schizophrenics' core psychopathology and in a technique which was non-directive and relied heavily upon evolution and change in a transference relationship. In contrast, the RAS therapists placed more importance on hereditary factors in the aetiology of schizophrenia and believed that these factors led to unmodifiable aspects of the schizophrenic patients' psychopathology. They also believed in a treatment approach which was directive and involved the formation of a relationship (Frosch et al. 1983).

Conceptualization of Treatment Strategies. It seems important to overcome the assumption of competition between therapeutic modalities and to design studies so that optimal combinations of therapeutic strategies can be assessed. If investigators limit their designs to simple drugs-versus-psychotherapy trials, interactions between treatments will not be discovered and understood. It is also possible that individual psychotherapy alone is not enough. It is also possible that insight-oriented, reflective and interpretative individual psychotherapy does not help schizophrenic patients (Gunderson et al. 1984). Combining family therapy and individual psychotherapy might be an alternative, but this has not yet been systematically studied. There is evidence that family therapy plus neuroleptic drugs together is more beneficial than one of them alone (Falloon et al. 1982; Goldstein and Kopeikin 1981).

References

Bookhammer RS (1966) A five-year clinical follow-up of schizophrenics treated by Rosen's direct analysis. Am J Psychiatry 123:602–604

Carpenter WT Jr (1984) A perspective on the psychotherapy of schizophrenia project. Schizophrenia Bull 10:599–603

Carpenter WT Jr, Barko JJ, Evans MSC (1983) Multivariate statistics and meaning in the study of psychopathology: Focus on a specific problem. Schizophrenia Bull 9:1–5

Fairweather GW, Simon R, Gebhard ME et al. (1960) Relative effectiveness of psychotherapeutic programs: a multicriteria comparison of four programs for three different patient groups. Psychological Monographs 74 (5):1–26

Falloon IRH, Boyd JL, McGill CW et al. (1982) Family management in the prevention of exacerbations of schizophrenia: a controlled study. N Engl J Med 306:1437–1440

Frosch JP, Gunderson JG, Weiss R, Frank A (1983) Therapists who treat schizophrenic patients: characterization. In: Stierlin H, Wynne LC, Wirsching M (eds) Psychosocial intervention in schizophrenia. Springer, Berlin Heidelberg New York Tokyo, pp 169–176

Goldberg SC, Schooler NR, Hogarty GE, Roper M (1977) Prediction of relapse in schizophrenic outpatients treated by drug and sociotherapy. Arch Gen Psychiatry 34:171–184

Goldstein MJ, Kopeikin HS (1981) Short- and long-term effect of combining drug and family therapy. In: Goldstein MJ (ed) New developments in interventions with families of schizophrenics. Jossey-Bass, San Francisco, pp 5–26

Grinspoon L, Ewalt JR, Shader RI (1972) Schizophrenia: pharmacotherapy and psychotherapy. Williams and Wilkins, Baltimore

Gunderson JG, Carroll A (1983) Clinical considerations from empirical research. In: Stierlin H, Wynne LC, Wirsching M (eds) Psychosocial intervention in schizophrenia. Springer, Berlin Heidelberg New York Tokyo, pp 125–142

Gunderson JG, Frank AD, Katz HM et al. (1984) Effect of psychotherapy in schizophrenia. II: Comparative outcome of two forms of treatment. Schizophrenia Bull 10:564–598

Heinrichs DW, Carpenter WT Jr (1981) The efficacy of individual psychotherapy: a perspective and review emphasizing controlled outcome studies. In: Arieti S, Brodie HK (eds) The American handbook of psychiatry, vol VII. Basic, New York, pp 586–613

Heinrichs DW, Carpenter WT Jr (1982) Psychotherapy of schizophrenic disorders. In: Grinspoon L (ed) Psychiatry 1982. American Psychiatric Press, Washington D.C., pp 154–166

Hogarty GE, Goldberg SC, Schooler NR et al. (1974) Drug and sociotherapy in the aftercare of schizophrenic patients: III. Adjustment of non-relapsed patients. Arch Gen Psychiatry 31:609–625

Karon L, VandenBos GR (1981) Schizophrenia: psychotherapy of schizophrenia: the treatment of choice. Aronson, New York

Katz HM, Frank A, Gunderson JG, Hamm D (1984) Psychotherapy of schizophrenia. What happens to treatment dropouts. J Nerv Ment Dis 172:326–331

Liem JH (1980) Family studies of schizophrenia: an update and commentary. In: Special Report: Schizophrenia 1980. National Institute of Mental Health, pp 82–108

May PRA (1968) Treatment of schizophrenia: a comparative study of five treatment methods. Science House, New York

May PRA, Tuma AH, Dixon WJ (1976a) Schizophrenia – a follow-up study of results of treatment. I. Design and other problems. Arch Gen Psychiatry 33:474–478

May PRA, Tuma AH, Yale C et al. (1976b) Schizophrenia – follow-up study of results of treatment. II. Hospital stay over two to five years. Arch Gen Psychiatry 33:481–486

May PRA, Tuma AH, Dixon WJ (1981) Schizophrenia – a follow-up study of the results of five forms of treatment. Arch Gen Psychiatry 38:776–784

Rogers CR, Gendlin RG, Kiesler DJ, Truax CB (eds) (1967) The therapeutic relationship and its impact: study of psychotherapy with schizophrenics. University of Wisconsin Press, Madison

Soskis DA (1972) A survey of psychiatric opinion on schizophrenia. Compr Psychiatry 13:573–580

Stanton AH, Gunderson JG, Knapp PH et al. (1984) Effects of psychotherapy in schizophrenia. I. Design and implementation of a controlled study. Schizophrenia Bull 10:520–563

Stierlin H, Wynne LC, Wirsching M (eds) (1983) Psychosocial intervention in schizophrenia. Springer, Berlin Heidelberg New York Tokyo

Strauss JS, Carpenter WT Jr (1981) Schizophrenia. Plenum, New York

Tienari P, Sorri A, Lahti I et al. (1985a) Interaction of genetic and psychosocial factors in schizophrenia. Acta Psychiatr Scand (Suppl 319):19–30

Tienari P, Sorri A, Lahti I et al. (1985b) The Finnish adoptive family study of schizophrenia. Yale J Biol Med 58:227–237

Wynne LC, Singer MT, Bartko JJ, Toohey ML (1977) Schizophrenics and their families: research on paternal communication. In: Tanner JM (ed) Developments in psychiatric research. Hodder and Stoughton, London, pp 245–286

Some Methodological Recommendations from the Hamburg Short Psychotherapy Comparison Experiment*

A.-E. MEYER[1]

Aim and Relevance

Our experiment compares psychodynamic conflict-centred time-limited therapy (PT) with client-centred therapy (CC), with special regard to outcome variables, content analyses and process scales. Sixty-eight patients of the psychosomatic department of Hamburg University Clinic were assigned at random to one of the two therapies. It is important to study the effectiveness of short-term psychotherapies as such, because they seem to be a solution to the continually increasing gap between the availability of and demand for psychotherapy. However, short-term psychotherapies are of course only useful when they are effective.

Sloane et al. (1975) compared PT with behaviour therapy and Grawe (1976) and Plog (1976) compared CC with behaviour therapy. We therefore decided to compare PT with CC to complete the comparisons. For a much more detailed description of our experiment, see Meyer (1981).

Intake Procedures

For 1½ years all patients who applied for an interview at our psychosomatic outpatient department and who were between 20 and 40 years and who claimed to have received no previous psychotherapy were invited to a testing session.

Of 286 patients invited, 72 did not come at all. The remaining 214 completed the psychological tests. Thereafter, these patients had to go through two intake assessments, the first being made by one of four client-centred therapists (a single session only), the other by one of four psychoanalysts (a minimum of two, rarely three sessions). There were drop-outs for various reasons (see Fig. 1).

In the next stage the remaining 177 patients were reported on individually and discussed in the "focus formulation seminar." (The reporting was done by

* Supported by grants from the Deutsche Forschungsgemeinschaft

[1] Abt. für Psychosomatik/Psychotherapie, Universitäts-Krankenhaus Eppendorf, II. Medizinische Klinik, Martinistraße 52, D-2000 Hamburg 20

Psychological Treatment of Mental Illness
Edited by R. J. Daly and E. A. Sand

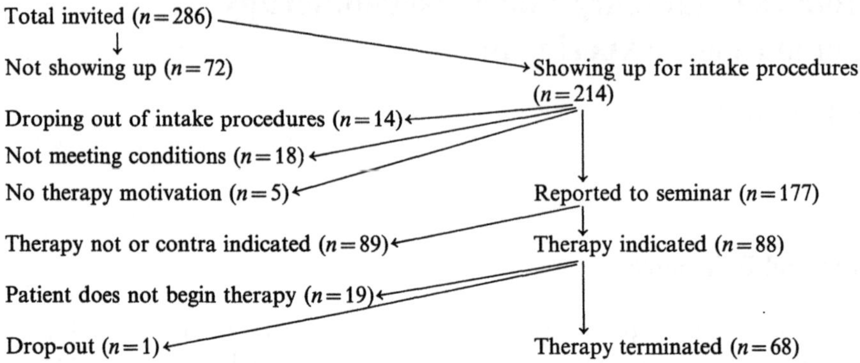

Fig. 1. Selection of patients

the analyst who had performed the intake interviews.) After focus formulation the seminar made a prognosis based on the focus and the other limiting conditions of our psychodynamic therapy. The guidelines for these prognostic predictions were taken from Malan (1963). There were four prognostic categories, good, medium, negative and contraindicated. Negative meant that the patient would neither profit nor suffer from our form of psychodynamic therapy and contraindicated implied that the patient would be harmed.

All of the patients with good and medium prognoses and half of those with negative prognoses were randomly assigned to CC or PT. For those patients assigned to CC the focus formulation was not given to the therapist so as not to confound the two treatments.

Selection Factors

We did a very careful study of selection factors (see Kimm et al. 1981), which yielded, among others, the following results. There was a preponderance of YAVIS (young, attractive, verbal, intelligent; Goldstein 1971) patients in our therapy sample. However, this was also true of the intake sample and was not heightened by the selection by our psychotherapists. Post hoc examination showed that the random assignments were truly random. The patients refusing therapy differed in two respects from those accepting therapy: they were less sick and less sophisticated. Special attention was given to the duration of symptoms or problems, because Eysenck (1961) postulated that spontaneous remission of symptoms is an exponential function of time, whereby 1 year after the start of symptoms 40% of the patients are much improved. This percentage rises to 65% after 2 years and reaches 90% after 5 years.

Although Eysenck's exponential remission theory is very probably false, it is interesting to see that in our sample 50% of the patients had been suffering

Table 1. Duration of problem

Time categories (year)	*n*	%
Less than 1	24	13.1
1– 2	26	14.0
2– 5	43	23.4
5–10	34	18.5
More than 10	57	31.0
Total	184	100.0

for 5 or more years when presenting themselves to our department (see Table 1). Thus, we treated a high proportion of chronic patients showing no tendendy towards remission.

Assessment Procedures

Since Maskelyne, director of the Greenwich Royal Observatory, reported in 1796 that he had fired his assistant because the latter's timing differed systematically from that of his superior, the problem of the personal equation has vexed science. In psychotherapy research this problem is even more prominent, because each witness has his or her own system of reference and measuring units. The patient rates his or her own pre–post change of life quality. The researcher compares within the group of research patients. The therapist judges with respect to similar patients he or she has treated and in regard to the therapy goals implicity or explicitly envisaged. Peers rate the changes in their relationship with the patient, and may find these negative if the patient has become more independent or self-assertive.

We know that there is neither an objective solution for nor a short cut to this Rashomon problem. Therefore we decided to engage as many witnesses as feasible and looked for congruence and disagreement and for the probable sources of both. In our Hamburg short psychotherapy comparison experiment, we questioned the patients using tests and interviews, the therapist gave a rating at the end of therapy, the intake interviewer also rated the two follow-ups, and a group of blind raters assessed the transcripts of the audiotaped follow-up interviews.

Our tests comprised subtests from the LPS (an intelligence test) and the following questionnaires:

1) The FPI, which is a test based on factor analysis having nine primary scales and three combined scales, the latter measuring "neuroticism," "extraversion" and "masculinity" (Fahrenberg and Selg 1970).
2) The GT which is also a test based on factor-analysis but its items were chosen to reflect psychoanalytic theory. The GT (Beckmann and Richter 1972) makes it possible to compare the real self with the ideal self. We also

used this test to determine the patient's view of the therapist and how this changed with time.

3) A third personality questionnaire, SAL, which is adapted from the Taylor Manifest Anxiety Scale (Spreen 1961).
4) The "symptom list" contained 152 items of neurotic or psychosomatic complaints, each rated for frequency and intensity. It was adapted from Pohlen (1972).

Control Group Design

For the evaluation of test results we strongly advocate the combination of own control group comparison with reference control group comparison. Own control compares, within the same patient, changes occurring during therapy with changes occurring during the waiting period. Reference control compares the changes occurring during therapy for patients treated immediately with the changes occurring during the waiting period in the above-mentioned non-identical sample. This combination has the following advantages: (a) own control uses a homogeneous sample but is subject to retest effects; with the reference control the contrary applies i.e. there is a heterogeneous sample but comparable retest effects. Thus the two procedures correct each other; (b) the two procedures allow for almost independent replication; differences found in both comparisons are accordingly more reliable; (c) every patient receives therapy and every patient takes part in the research.

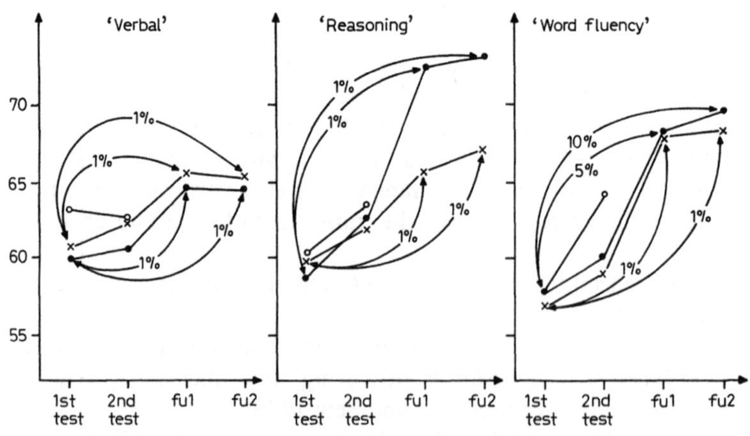

Fig. 2. Results with intelligence subtests of LPS. Reference control group comparison analysis of variance. *1st test*, pretherapy; *2nd test*, posttherapy; *fu1*, follow-up after 3 months; *fu2*, follow-up after 9 months. Percentage values indicate level of significance

Outcome Results for Different Variables

Some selected examples should illustrate our procedure. Reference control comparison showed that the gains in three intelligence subtests during therapy were not significantly superior to those during the waiting period, which also achieved sizeable gains (see Fig. 2). We conclude that the spectacular gains are not due to therapy but to retest effects engendered by practice. In reference control comparison the meanscore for "Sociability" (see Fig. 3) (a component of extraversion) increased significantly more in both therapies than during waiting. These gains were stable over the two follow-ups. Judging from own control comparison (see Fig. 4) this could be a retest effect for CC but not for PT. Considering the comparisons together, the results imply real gains for both therapies.

Similar examples can be found for the FPI scale "depression," where both reference and own Control showed a significant decrease for CC but not for PT (see Stuhr et al. 1981, Figs. 5 and 6, p. 149), and for "aggression" where both comparisons showed a heightening for PT but not for CC (see Stuhr et al. 1981, Figs. 3 and 4, p. 148).

Concerning our clinical ratings, we first analysed the blind group ratings of the transcribed follow-up interviews (see Meyer et al. 1981, Tables 2–4, pp. 203–205). For insight variables all significant differences implied a heightening for PT. This is probably not due to observer bias because in other respects CC emerged with superior ratings. We found that both therapies were equally effective with the main symptoms and CC was more effective for minor or secondary symptoms, although this success had almost vanished at the time of the second follow-up.

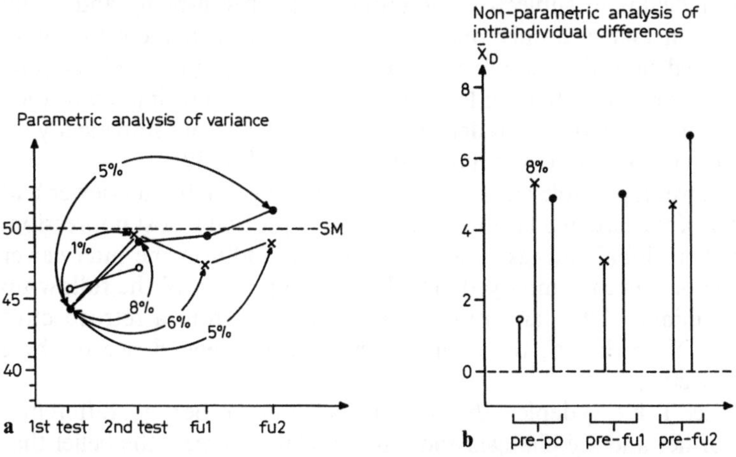

Fig. 3a, b. Reference control group comparison of "socialbility" (FPI scale 5). **a** o——o, waiting group; ×——×, immediate psychdynamic psychotherapy; ●——● immediate client-centred therapy; SM, standardization sample's mean; $\bar{x}_D$, arithmetic mean of intraindividual differences. **b** pre-po, $\bar{x}_D$ from first test to second test; pre-fu1, $\bar{x}_D$ from pretherapy to follow-up 1; pre-fu2, $\bar{x}_D$ from pretherapy to follow-up 2

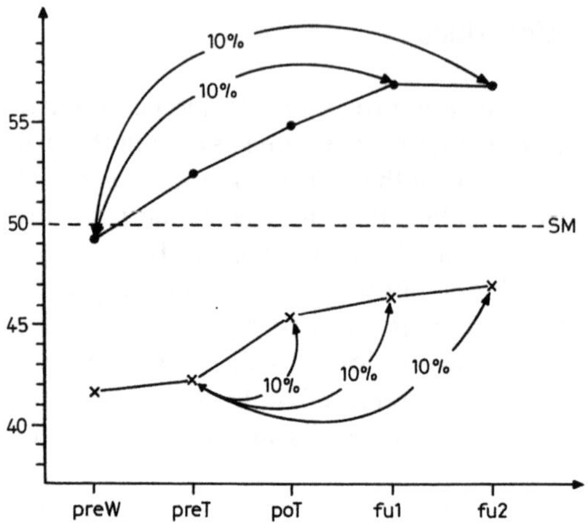

Fig. 4. Own control group comparison of "sociability" (FPI scale 5). SM, standardization sample's mean, ×——×, sample who waited for and then received psychodynamic psychotherapy; ●——●, sample who waited for and then received client-cenred therapy, preW, waiting period; preT, pretherapy; poT, post-therapy

The Integration of Outcome Variables

The test scales used were constructed to be statistically independent, but this was not so for our clinical ratings. Therefore, we used factor analysis as a first step. Four factors were extracted and varimax rotated for simple structure. These four factors explained 47.9% of the total variance (for a complete description see Deneke et al. 1987).

On factor 1 (see Table 2), explaining 22% of the total variance, all three witness groups (blind group, the four interviewers and the patients) agreed that the patient is feeling better, has less symptoms and is better able to cope. We called factor 1 "gains in subjective symptom-oriented well-being and social competence." On factor 2 only one group of witnesses, namely the blind group, converged on only one phenomenon, namely "insight." This is quite disconcerting as we found that our four interviewers' insight ratings converged on factor 3. Thus, the two groups delivered ratings which were statistically independent from each other (for details see Deneke et al. 1987).

There are several possible causes of this discrepancy. Each interviewer had seen a quarter of the patients face to face and had a pre and a post impression, but made rather global ratings in a short time. In addition the interviewer knew the type of therapy employed. The blind group rated all the follow-up transcripts in minute detail and rated therapy changes from a retrospective point of view. Nevertheless, the complete statistical independence of these judgments is peculiar.

Factor 4 (see Table 3) depicts the patient's belief that others act differently toward him or her and see changes and – to a certain degree – the belief that he or she did change. This is statistically independent from the "feeling better" and "able to manage his or her life" which load on factor 1 (see Table 2). However, the blind group rated "attitude of others toward patient" equally on factor 1 (see item 24 in Table 2). In this case we find the patients' differentiation

Table 2. Factor 1: gains in subjective symptom-oriented wellbeing and social competence

Variables	Witness	a
16. Symptom 1[a]	b.g.	0.68
17. Symptom 2	b.g.	0.81
18. Symptom 3	b.g.	0.80
19. Symptom 4	b.g.	0.76
20. Symptom 5	b.g.	0.53
21. Symptom 6	b.g.	0.57
22. Overall rating for symptoms	b.g.	0.92
23. Attitudes and behaviour to others	b.g.	0.81
24. Attitudes and behaviour of others to the patient	b.g.	0.72
25. Change of the life practice	b.g.	0.61
26. Ego-restriction	b.g.	0.85
28. Subjective wellbeing	b.g.	0.93
29. Attitude to own self	b.g.	0.87
30. Overall rating of all changes	b.g.	0.91
31. Patient feeling therapy helped	b.g. (pat.)	0.51
Feeling better	pat.	0.77
Able to manage his or her life	pat.	0.77
Social progress	int.	0.57
Reduction of the symptoms	int.	0.53
Subjective wellbeing	int.	0.65
Symptom 1	int.	0.44

[a] Graduation 1–6 according to the subjective importance of the symptom. Abbreviations: a, factor loading; b.g., blind group follow-up rating; pat., patient self-judgement; int., judgement of the interviewers.

Table 3. Factor 4: change in self plus interpersonal relation (judged by the patient)

Variable	Witness	a
"I feel that others have changed towards me"	pat.	0.83
"I think that others see me changed"	pat.	0.79
"I have changed myself by the therapy, somehow"	pat.	0.55

Abbreviations: a, loading on factor V; pat., patient.

more plausible and think that they are in a better position to judge such often subtle changes. We presume that the patients did not articulate these beliefs clearly enough in the interviews.

We have only described the integration of clinical outcome ratings here. For details of the integration of test results and the overall integration of both sets of data, see Stuhr and Meyer (1987) and Meyer and Stuhr (1987).

Unsolved Problems

The Timing of Follow-Ups. Grawe (1975) found in his study that, at the end of therapy, behaviour therapy was clearly superior in outcome to CC. At a 4-

Table 4. Correlations of factor scores (of individual patients) from the two follow-ups

	Total	CC	PT
F_1	0.41*	0.39	0.21
F_2	0.51**	0.69**	0.22
F_3	0.65**	0.89**	0.40*
F_4	0.69**	0.84**	0.25

Abbreviations: F, factor; CC, sample with client centred therapy; PT, sample with psychodynamic therapy.
* $P<0.05$, ** $P<0.01$.

month follow-up these differences had vanished because CC patients had made additional gains in the meantime, but behaviour therapy patients had remained stable. Our test results indicated a temporary relapse at a follow-up 3 months after therapy ended, especially for PT, with a regain at a follow-up 9 months after therapy (Stuhr et al. 1981, p. 194).

Table 4 shows that the patients' factor scores are not stable from the 3-month to the 9-month follow-up: this implies factor 1 (see Table 2) for both CC and PT, and factors 2 and 4 for PT only. If such findings are replicated by other authors, they would show that the timing of the follow-ups is important in determining the observed outcome.

The Problem of Pre–Post Differences. Pre–post differences have statistically undesirable features. Mathematical deduction shows that when pre and post measurements are uncorrelated, their difference correlates +0.70 with the diminuend (= pre) and −0.70 with the subtractor (= post.). Our own Monte Carlo simulations with random numbers show that this correlation can be as great as ±0.80. Another difficulty is regression to the mean, superimposed by the "normalizing" effect of therapy. Hopefully, the law of initial values does not apply to pre–post results. However, existing attempts and recommendations to partial out these interacting influences (see Zielke 1982) do not convince me.

Whole Sample Versus Taxometric Analyses. Whole-sample comparisons can be clinically misleading. They camouflage the small percentage (2%–3%, occasionally 7%; see Mintz 1977, Table 2) of patients who deteriorate under psychotherapy instead of making them identifiable and protecting them from this form of therapy. Equally, they camouflage individual therapy goals. The mean extraversion score is usually significantly heightened after pschotherapy. For a majority of neurotic patients, who are insecure and feel guilty and anxious in social contacts, this is indeed a desired and acceptable change. However, there is a minority of "acting out" or "hysterical" patients for whom the contrary is true. If therapy achieves a lowering of "extraversion" for this subgroup, this effect can either disappear or can lower the whole sample's difference (and/or heighten the variance of the post measurements) so that the comparison may become statistically non-significant.

I have argued (Meyer 1985) that while single-case studies are a poor alternative because they may not be representative, a good alternative can be found in taxometrics. By this I mean all procedures that group patients into taxa by virtue of their reciprocal similarity. These procedures are mainly the various cluster methods, but also include Q factor analysis and configuration frequency analysis (Lienert and Rey 1981). Our own results with taxometric procedures will soon be evaluated.

References

Beckmann D, Richter H-E (1972) Der Giessen-Test (GT). Huber, Bern

Deneke F-W, Stuhr U, Meyer A-E, Burzig G (1987) Factor analytic reintegration of clinical outcome ratings. Psychother Psychosom (to be published)

Eysenck HJ (1961) The effects of psychotherapy. In: Eysenck HJ (ed) Handbook of abnormal psychology. Basic Books, New York, pp 697–725

Fahrenberg J, Selg J (1970) Freiburger Persönlichkeits-Inventar FPI. Hogrefe, Göttingen

Goldstein (1971) Psychotherapeutic attraction. Pergamon, New York

Grawe K (1976) Differentielle Psychotherapie. I. Huber, Bern

Kimm HJ, Bolz W, Meyer A-E (1981) The patient sample: overt and covert selection factors and prognostic predictions. Psychother Psychosom 35:96–109

Lienert GA, Rey ER (1981) Die Konfigurationsfrequenzanalyse. XV. Typenexploration und -inferenz. Z Klin Psychol Psychother 29:209–215

Malan D (1963) A study of brief psychotherapy. Tavistock, London

Maskelyne N (1796) Astronomical observations made on the royal observatory at Greenwich, vol 3, p 339

Meyer A-E (ed) (1981) The Hamburg short psychotherapy comparison experiment. Karger, Basel

Meyer A-E (1985) Grundlagen, Konzepte und Methoden der Psychotherapie-Forschung. Verh Dtsch Ges Inn Med 91

Meyer A-E, Bolz W, Stuhr U, Burzig G (1981) Outcome results by clinical evaluation based on the blind group ratings. Psychother Psychosom 35:199–207

Meyer A-E, Stuhr U (1987) Integration of clinical with test outcome data. Psychother Pschosom (to be published)

Mintz J (1977) The role of the therapist in assessing psychotherapy outcome. In: Gurman AS, Razin AM (eds) Effective psychotherapy. Pergamon, Oxford

Plog U (1976) Differentielle Psychotherapy, vol 2. Huber, Bern

Pohlen M (1972) Gruppenanalyse. Vandenhoek and Ruprecht, Göttingen

Sloane RB, Staples PR, Christel AH, Yorkston NJ, Wipple K (1975) Psychotherapy versus behaviour therapy. Harvard University Press, Cambridge

Spreen O (1961) Konstruktion einer Skala zur Messung der manifesten Angst in experimentellen Untersuchungen. Psychol Forsch 26:205–223

Stuhr U, Meyer A-E, Bolz W (1981) Outcome results in psychological tests. Psychother Psychosom 35:138–198

Stuhr U, Meyer A-E (1987) Differential change patterns in tests (to be published)

Zielke M (1982) Probleme und Ergebnisse der Veränderungsmessung. In: Zielke M (ed) Diagnostik in der Psychotherapie. Kohlhammer, Stuttgart, pp 41–59

Experimental Design in Behavioural Psychotherapy

I. M. MARKS[1]

There is no single methodology for the study of behavioural treatment, just as there is no single methodology for any research. It all depends on the questions one is asking, and a variety of approaches are needed for different issues. I will describe a selection of some of the designs that have been used in the past and some of the issues that have been raised, and will then suggest where we might go in the future.

There is a use both for single-case designs and for group designs. The phase of the research when single-case designs are useful is early in exploration of a question. Group designs, which are more expensive, come later in the research process. Single-case designs can only be of a pilot nature because we never know how representative single cases are. Group designs, if they are well done, are more definitive and can lead to firmer conclusions. With single-case designs one is always left wondering, no matter how good they are, whether that case was atypical. An advantage of a single-case design is that one needs few patients. Many patients are needed for group designs, and in uncommon conditions especially, it could take many years to complete the design. The cost of single-case studies is generally small, but group designs of most kinds, on the other hand, are usually expensive. In Britain the cost of our drug-behavioural studies using factorial designs is about £ 100000 per question, so one has to be sure the question is right. Also, the time for completion of single-case designs, in general, is much quicker than for group studies.

What kind of information can we get from single-case designs? Professor Gelder and I long ago studied a transvestite patient. By appropriate manipulation within a single case one can get some idea of whether one's treatment procedure is effecting change across physiological and attitudinal variables. The transvestite was asked to imagine himself dressing in women's panties, women's pyjamas, skirt, blouse and slip, and we measured the time it took him to obtain an image of each of these garments – the latency. Each time he reported that he got the image, he was shocked. The order in which each set of fantasies was shocked was reflected by the order in which the latency to obtain the fantasy of that garment rose. It became more and more difficult to get that particular fantasy, but not other fantasies, e.g. at one phase although he could not imagine women's panties he could still imagine women's pyjamas. The

[1] Institute of Psychiatry, Maudsley Hospital, London SE5 8AF, United Kingdom

Psychological Treatment of Mental Illness
Edited by R. J. Daly and E. A. Sand

erections were measured with an instrument devised by Dr Bancroft, who was working with us at the time. The patient had erections to photographs of nude women, and to touching women's panties, slips, skirts and pyjamas. Before treatment he got erections rapidly to all of these but as fantasies were successively shocked, the erections to the objects disappeared in the same order. On semantic differential attitudes, too, there were corresponding changes in the same order. At the beginning all women's garments were rated as very friendly and pleasant, but at the end of the first series of shocks to women's panties, the attitude reversed to become negative. So this single-case study yielded concordant changes in fantasies, in erections and in attitude which indicated that at least the total therapeutical procedure had something to do with the change, though one cannot say for certain that it was the shock; for that we need further controls. For each question we have to tailor our design to fit the problem.

There are studies intermediate between single and group designs. Stravinsky, Yule and I gave social skills training for social skills deficits in a multiple-baseline design. One series of social activities were treated and another series were left untreated. Systematically for several patients, the first social task was treated after an initial variable period of baseline measurement. Other social activities were treated later and several remained untreated. Whenever social skills training for a particular social activity was introduced, that activity began to improve highly significantly, whereas untreated tasks remain unchanged. In multiple-baseline work it is regrettably not customary to carry out statistical tests of significance. One can, however, do a variety of statistical tests across the contingency (the point at which treatment began) and across other time periods to show that in fact it is the introduction of treatment rather than time or just being in an experiment that is important.

After completing the multiple-baseline design all patients entered a group design. They were assigned at random either to social skills training by itself or to social skills training with cognitive modification. They were treated for several months and then followed up for 6 months. Improvement in both groups was highly significant from start to finish, but adding cognitive therapy added nothing to outcome. (Another study showed that cognitive therapy did not augment improvement of agoraphobics from exposure.) On completing the multiple-baseline design patients then entered a factorial design which found that there was no difference between treatments. We also answered an important point about process as well as outcome. We measured the number of irrational beliefs that the patients had, and found that these diminished to the same extent whether or not cognitive modification was added to the social skills training. If we changed the behaviour, then attitude change followed as well. One does not need to deal with the irrational beliefs in order to effect improvement; change the behaviour and the beliefs change in turn.

Let us turn to a different type of group study – long-term follow-ups. Inevitably we have no control over what happens to patients once they are discharged but there is every point in following them up over several years and comparing the follow-up outcomes from different studies. It is especially useful if the studies have used identical measuring instruments. As an example, obsessive-compulsive ritualizers were treated in London by Rachman, Hodgson and myself, in Philadelphia by Foa and in Athens by Boulougouris and Rabavilas. We all used identical scales and the patients had a similar severity of ritual behaviour at the start. The treatment was exposure in vivo with self-imposed response prevention, and patients were followed up for various periods of time. The longest follow-up was the Greek study, 3 years; that of the London study was 2 years and of the Philadelphia study 15 months. It is interesting how congruent improvement was over follow-up in the three studies, both in symptoms and in work adjustment. Long-term follow up studies of this kind unfortunately are still far too few, though they are a critical issue in cost-benefit analysis, as I will discuss later.

Let us take another example of a factorial design. We were interested in learning whether therapist contact was necessary for improvement to occur during exposure in vivo. Exposure treatment simply brings the patient into contact with the stimulus which evokes phobias or rituals and persuades him or her to remain there until the phobias or rituals subside. We assigned patients at random to one of three conditions. In one condition they were simply given an instruction manual to read – my book *Living With Fear* (McGraw-Hill 1980), which has a self-help chapter. They were simply told to read the book and follow its instructions. The second group had to sit at a computer terminal and to interact with it (it had been programmed with self-help instructions from *Living With Fear*) and the third group had a psychiatrist giving the same instructions for exposure. All treatment was self-exposure and the total contact of the psychiatrist, with the patient was 40 min in the book group, about 1 hour in the computer group, and 3 hours in the therapist group.

Our initial hypothesis was that the more interaction there was with the therapeutic agent, the better the outcome would be. We predicted that the order of improvement would be best in the psychiatrist-instructed group, next in the computer-instructed group which has some flexibility, and last in the book-instructed group. Rather to our surprise, all three groups of patients improved highly significantly and retained this improvement for up to 6 months, so our hypothesis that some kind of interaction with the therapeutic agent would enhance the outcome was not borne out. Just giving a self-treatment manual was sufficient.

Perhaps we should have given them some other book to read, a Len Deighton thriller or The Bible, as a different control. However, there is a great deal of other research suggesting that exposure in some form is the key ingredient in this therapy, and that is why we did not test the exposure hypothesis in this study. Despite the tight design, and interesting results, there remain issues we have to consider that this study didn't answer. Two of the patients in the book-treated group had in fact bought *Living With Fear* in a bookstore in London, but did not follow its instructions until the therapist told them to do so. Clearly there are motivational variables we have to take into account that are not dealt with by a design of this kind.

To answer all questions in a particular area, one needs a variety of designs. Early in the development of exposure therapy for obsessive-compulsives, we found a patient who was involved in a marital battle with her husband. A single-case experiment was performed (in collaboration with Dr. Richard Stern). She had had much exposure therapy, to no avail. We then decided to try an alternative approach, marital contract therapy, where the patient and her husband would give one another agreed rewards, and found that within a couple of sessions this couple had become like lovebirds on honeymoon. The contracts were that the husband had to build all the kitchen furniture that she had previously requested. The wife agreed to engage in sex again – they hadn't had sex for a year. By the second session they were having sex again every night and the kitchen contained furniture that the husband had built, and he was also talking with her again for the first time. Surprisingly, the rituals diminished for the first time. Though extensive exposure had had no effect, with contract therapy the patient suddenly started to improve and this was maintained until 12 weeks follow up.

We thought that maybe this supported the idea that rituals kept the marriage together. We therefore embarked on a controlled study. That was a very sobering thing to do.

The design was executed by John Cobb, Richard Stern and myself. Patients were randomly assigned either to marital therapy or to exposure therapy. Both therapies were with couples, the marital therapy being of the contract therapy variety; there then followed a buffer intervening period of 3 months, after which the reverse therapy was given, in a crossover design. We did not want to do a crossover design because it confounds long-term follow up, but being short of suitable patients we were forced to opt for the next-best option.

The outcome of this group study differed from that of the single-case study. If anything, it was the reverse. In 11 couples the exposure therapy improved the rituals more than the marital therapy did. When patients switched from marital to exposure therapy they improved further; moreover the marital problems improved more with exposure therapy than they did with marital therapy. So we have to be careful. We cannot extrapolate much from single cases. The ideas generated by single cases must be tested in larger group designs.

We looked again at the issue of the relationship between marital outcome and phobias in another study, and found that although the patients improved in their phobias their marital adjustment tended to remain unchanged. The phobias of those with initially good marriages did significantly better, but the marriages remained the same. The idea that in some way phobias keep the partners together did not hold up.

We will now consider an incomplete crossover-controlled study of behavioural psychotherapy for neurotics in primary care. The behavioural psychotherapy was done by a nurse therapist. The comparison group was patients randomly assigned to continued routine treatment by the general practitioner for 1 year. The results for the first year showed that nurse therapist-treated cases having behavioural treatment improved significantly more than did the routine treated cases. The drop outs whom we could follow up did not change significantly. After a year, we offered behavioural treatment to the patients treated by the general practitioner who had not improved (the majority). These patients now getting behavioural psychotherapy for the first time then improved, and as far as we could follow them up they retained their improvement.

I wish to address the issue of cost-benefit analysis. In a previous pilot study of nurse therapists which was uncontrolled, we looked at the benefits to the patient and health service and at all the costs involved in treatment. We found that the internal rate of return was very negative until improvement continued into the third year of follow up; at that point it became very positive, i.e. we started getting "money" back, in purely monetary terms. This disregarded the value of relieved anxiety, decreased depression, and so on.

We then decided to do a controlled study, some of the clinical results of which were described above. We did the same thing as in the pilot study. We looked at the change in the care utilization patterns in the year before treatment compared with 1 year after trial entry. A number of non-significant changes favoured the behavioural psychotherapy group (the nurse therapy group). The change was significant for the number of visits to the general practitioner. Overall, the nurse therapy group reduced its costs slightly while the untreated patients increased their costs.

The benefit-to-cost ratio became greater than one towards the end of the second year of follow up. From the end of the second year the community started to get it's money back on the therapeutic investment in terms of salaries. This is in agreement with the results of the pilot study. The duration of benefits over follow up is critical in deciding whether or not the tangible benefits are worthwhile.

Finally, these investigations suggest the need for more long-term follow ups of clinical studies. Controlled studies are all very well but far too many of them in the behavioural and drug field have follow up periods that are too brief for us to draw cost-benefit conclusions. A further point is important. Comparison across different studies in Europe, America and elsewhere is confounded by the wide variety of different instruments for measurement. There may be some point in European and American research organizations setting up a common measurement depository for the various psychological instruments that are being used, so that anybody wanting to use a given instrument can turn to that central clearing house. If we had a standard facility of this kind, it might encourage researchers to use more standard instruments and some of the problems of comparing different studies might be reduced.

Evaluation of Behavioural Treatments

B. Samuel-Lajeunesse[1] and M. Agathon

Introduction

One of the advantages of behaviour therapy is that it deals with tèchniques derived from experimental psychology. Thus, therapists have always been concerned with the assessment of the results of their treatment and have developed many methods and strategies to test its effectiveness.

In 1972 Kanfer pointed out that the goals and scope of behaviour therapy are to obtain "a specific observable class of behaviour rather than a change in the personality structure of the patient." Despite these limitations in goals and scope, behaviour therapists still remain unsatisfied with the measures available. As stressed by Lazarus (1976), therapists ought to include more of parameters in their assessments. In specific fields such as phobias, attempts have been made to obtain a general estimation of both behavioural and clinical developments (e.g. Gelder 1967; Watchell 1977; Emmelkamp 1979). However, one of the main criticisms which has been made of behaviour therapy when evaluating outcome is, as stressed by Lamontagne (1980), that studies "seldom refer to a clinical picture but focus only on modifiable symptoms." We believe that the combined efforts of psychiatrists with their clinical experience and of psychotherapists with their specific approach might help to elaborate new ways of assessing the outcome of psychotherapeutic treatments.

As a clinician in a teaching department one of us has suggested to both therapists of the psychoanalytic unit and to those of the behaviour unit that they combine their efforts in order to elaborate new tools for the evaluation of results of psychotherapy. This proposal has been well received by behaviour therapists but not by psychoanalysts. Therefore, the present study attempts to appreciate the differences between clinical and behavioural assessment whatever the technique used.

All studies have pointed out (Sloane 1979) that the correlations between the assessments of the clinician, the behaviour therapist and the patient are low. As expected, the most favourable assessments of the effects of psychotherapy are those of the behaviour therapist. In this study, independently of other phobic scales, we used six-point scales rating the following factors: the

[1] Clinique des Maladies Mentales et de l'Encéphale, CHR Sainte-Anne, Université Paris V, 100, rue de la Santé, F-75674 Paris Cedex 14

Psychological Treatment of Mental Illness
Edited by R. J. Daly and E. A. Sand

Clinique des Maladies Mentales et de l'Encéphale
Unité de Thérapie Comportementale
Auto-Evaluation

Name: .... Date: ....

I. *Symptomatology*

A. Which are the three main symptoms bothering you? (please note the score from 1 to 6)

	1	2	3	4	5	6
1)						
2)						
3)						

B. Do you presently feel anxious?						
C. Do you presently feel depressed?						

II. *Handicap*

– Do you have any trouble in the following fields?

– professional life						
– social life..........................						
– family life						
– marital life						
– sexual life						

III. How do you feel about your state of health since the beginning of the treatment?

☐ – much improved or cured
☐ – improved
☐ – without change
☐ – slightly worse
☐ – worse

Fig. 1. The self-assessment questionnaire given to patients (translation)

four main symptoms or behaviours on which the treatment is focused; general anxiety; depressed feelings; and impairment of professional, leisure and sexual activity, and family difficulties.

Overall results were rated on a five-points scale. Assessments were made before and 4 months after the beginning of the treatment, independently by the patients themselves (see Fig. 1), by a psychiatrist acting as an independent observer and by the behaviour therapists. The psychiatrist did not interfere with the behavioural treatment, but administration of any drugs was under his control.

The study deals with 33 outpatients including 20 suffering from phobic troubles and four with obsessive disorders. Diagnosis was made by the psychiatrist according to the INSERM classification as follows: 29 neurotic states including 20 phobic neuroses, four obsessive neuroses, one neurotic depression, and four unclassified neurotic states; four cases of neurotic symptoms accompanying psychiatric disorders, including three manic-depressive psychoses of the depressive type and one chronic schizophrenia of the schizoaffective type.

In order to point out some problems that arise in assessments of behavioural treatments, we shall present some results of this study.

Results

Symptoms or Behaviours (Table 1). There was a high correlation between the patients' and the psychiatrist's ratings at the second assessment. The correlation at the first assessment was, however, not significant. This could be explained by symptoms being rated independently and freely by both raters. Initially the same symptoms may be given different labels, but later the psychiatrist may be more sensitive to the behaviours focused on during treatment.

Ratings by patients and behaviour therapists evidently focused much more on the same semiology, and there was also a surprisingly high correlation between the ratings of the psychiatrist and the therapists.

Anxiety (Table 2). In the initial assessment there were no correlations between the ratings of the patients and the therapists or between the psychiatrist and the therapists, as could be expected given the difficulties in assessment of anxiety. Better correlations were found at the second assessment, which could be explained by the lower anxiety level at that time.

Impairment. The best correlations of ratings were found for the second assessment (Table 3). The differences between the ratings of patients and therapists were initially high, being very high because therapists are more focused on the behaviours which are to be treated.

Overall Evolution. The best correlations of ratings were found between the patients' and therapists' ratings (Table 4).

Table 1. Correlations (R) between ratings of symptoms at two independent assessments

	Initial	Final
Patient/psychiatrist	NS	0.63***
Patient/therapist	0.34**	0.56***
Psychiatrist/therapist	0.34*	0.44***

* $P<0.05$, ** $P<0.025$, *** $P<0.01$.

Table 2. Correlations (R) between ratings of anxiety at two independent assessments

	Initial	Final
Patient/psychiatrist	0.76***	0.64***
Patient/therapist	NS	0.41***
Psychiatrist/therapist	NS	0.38**

** $P<0.025$, *** $P<0.01$.

Table 3. Correlations (R) between ratings of impairment at two independent assessments

	Initial	Final
Patient/psychiatrist	0.59***	0.73***
Patient/therapist	0.30*	0.69***
Psychiatrist/therapist	NS	0.73***

* $P<0.05$, *** $P<0.01$.

Table 4. Correlations (R) between ratings of overall evolution

	Initial	Final
Patient/psychiatrist	×	0.82***
Patient/therapist	×	0.53***
Psychiatrist/therapist	×	0.57***

*** $P<0.01$.

Comments

There was a better correlation at both assessments between the ratings of patients and psychiatrist than between behaviour therapists and patients. From a theoretical point of view the idea of an independent rater seems reasonable. However, in this study it could be said that the psychiatrist was involved in the therapeutic process even if he was ignorant of the therapeutic technique used. Moreover, the psychiatrist's ratings were based only on the comments of patients; under these conditions it seems difficult to assert that the psychiatrist really was acting as an independent rater.

The ratings themselves raise some questions. Some methodological problems are that mean scores were used and that comparison was made between ratings given at the same time and not done between the ratings given at the two assessments. The main problem is that symptoms or behaviours were rated independently of the situation in which they occurred and without consideration of the cognitions linked to them.

In order to obtain better assessments, especially in behaviour treatments, we suggest that all ratings be done, if possible, during treatment and that their cognitive aspects be considered. An independent observer is useful but in many studies, as here, this independence is debatable, even if the observers are students watching video-tapes. A problem with the use video-tapes is that they may be unable to collect all the data needed for the assessment.

We need data on the outcome of various psychotherapies as well as on the processes of the treatments. The most interesting ratings of outcome are those done by the patient, because whatever the underlaying theories of the psychotherapist, the patient's satisfaction is the main aim of treatment. We also need data on the results of various psychotherapeutic techniques, as has been done for biological treatments.

Studies of outcome seem to be more useful, at this time, than studies on the processes of psychotherapies. These studies could be done either on simple cases or on patient groups – it is mainly a matter of what funds are available. The two methods are complementary, and their promotion is necessary despite some methodological and economical problems. At present surprisingly few studies have been published on the treatment of anxiety disorders. Multicentre studies of anxious patients treated with psychological techniques, drugs or placebo could perhaps be initiated by an international organization.

References

Emmelkamp MPG (1979) The behavioural study of clinical phobics. In: Hersen M, Eisler RM, Miller PM (eds) Progress in behaviour modification. Academic, New York

Gelder MG, Marks IM, Wolff HH, Clarke B (1967) Desensitization and psychotherapy in the treatment of phobic states: a controlled enquiry. Br J Psychiatry 113:53–73

Kanfer FH (1972) Assessments of behaviour modification. J Pers Assess 36:418–423

Lamontagne Y (1980) Initiation à la recherche en psychologie clinique et en psychiatrie. Edisem, Québec

Lazarus, AA (1976) Multimodal behaviour therapy. Springer, Berlin Heidelberg New York

Samuel-Lajeunesse B, Agathon M (1982) Therapeutic results of 33 neurotic patients. Clinical and behavioural assessments. Act Nerv Super 24:119–127

Sloane RS, Staples FR, Cristol PH, Yorkston N, Whipple R (1975) Psychotherapy versus behavior therapy. Harvard University Press, Cambridge

Watchel BE (1977) Psychoanalysis and behaviour therapy: toward an integration. Basic, New York

Special Design Approaches to Small Groups and Mixed Treatments

K. G. Götestam[1]

Introduction

In the area of psychological treatments of mental illness, research strategies and experimental designs have become more and more emphasized. For drugs the Food and Drug Administration and other national controlling boards have developed sets of standards determining how a new (drug) treatment should be tested. This has not so far been the case with psychotherapy. The evaluation of improvements to psychotherapy, however, is in great need of such standards, and on our way towards control by the national health authorities of the effectiveness of our therapy, we have been eagerly working to improve the scientific evaluative instruments.

Although this development has for some time been heavily dominated by a behavioural orientation, this need not be so. Some behavioural assessments could also be used for psychodynamic approaches to treatment and, more importantly, some of the experimental designs could be applied to the evaluation of psychodynamic psychotherapy.

In this paper some special design approaches will be presented, with special emphasis on small groups, which are a typical problem in psychotherapy research, and on mixed treatment, which is a rather overlooked method to test two or more therapy techniques (medical and psychological for example) simultaneously. In this paper examples will be taken from our own research, which, because of the lack of psychodynamic research already mentioned, will be mostly of a behavioural character. Several handbooks exist on this subject, and the one by Kazdin (1980) is recommended.

The Small Group Problem

In psychotherapy research, as in research on other therapies, one is often dealing with only a small group of patients, which makes research inconvenient and difficult, and thus often not done. This fact, which makes it difficult to perform conventional group studies, may have several explanations.

[1] University of Trondheim, Department of Psychiatry and Behavioural Medicine, Östmarka Hospital, N-7001 Trondheim, Norway

Psychological Treatment of Mental Illness
Edited by R. J. Daly and E. A. Sand

Patients Not Accessible. Either the patients with the specific problem to be studied do not exist in large numbers, or, more often, they are not present in one place or one area, and are thus not available to one researcher or research group.

Exclusion Criteria. When there is a large enough sample, the exclusion and inclusion criteria often restrict the group further, so again it is too small for a group study.

Possible Participants Unwilling to Participate. When patients are recruited for a study, they may have little or lose motivation "to be studied," and therefore may be unwilling to participate or they drop out during the study.

Refusal to be Randomized for Treatment. Another problem is that patients may be unwilling to be randomly assigned to participate in a particular therapy. To be useful for study, they should be willing to accept two different treatments, and then be randomly assigned to one of them, without any choice themselves. Again, this may lead to refusal to participate or drop out from the study.

Legal and Ethical Restrictions. There are legal restrictions on performing a clinical study. The medical authorities may in fact oppose a study of the effect of a treatment they believe effective, even if the effectiveness has not been scientifically proven. There are also ethical restrictions with regards to control-group procedures. Non-treatment participation should not result in abstinence from effective treatment for too long.

Limited Resources. To conduct a clinical trial of a new drug, one needs resources such as funding, staff, equipment and hospital beds. As a psychotherapy trial often takes more time than a drug trial, psychotherapy needs even greater research resources if it is to be realistic.

Time Restrictions. In a clinical setting it is often difficult to find enough time for research. This is especially true when large patient groups are compared over long time periods.

Conventional Solutions

Conventionally there have been two strategies to solve the above problems, the multicentre study, and the anecdotal case study. Both of these strategies, however, suffer from severe shortcomings.

The Multicentre Solution. The multicentre study may often be a solution to some of the above-mentioned problems. In many instances it is an acceptable or even a good solution, but there are two kinds of problems often connected with this approach. One is that the design is not sufficiently well developed and supervised during the study (a recent exception is the study of Elkin et al. 1985). Another shortcoming is that the number of patients may be increased at the expense of the stringency of the experimental design. A poor design with 20 patients does not get better if 100 patients are tested!

The Anecdotal Case Study. A more traditional solution to the small group problem has been to make a case study with an anecdotal rather than an experimental approach. This has certainly been of vast importance in the area of psychotherapy, first to present a new idea (and research challenge) for a treatment approach, and secondly to implant and spread the idea, i.e. with a more educational aim. It should be noted, however, that the anecdotal case study allows alternative explanations to the one expressed by the therapist, some of which are as follows: (1) coincidental events, i.e. some factor other than the therapy, can parallel therapy and cause the effect observed; (2) time alone can often heal the illness, in what we call spontaneous (i.e.cause unknown) healing; (3) the assessments may be reactive in themselves and cause an improvement; (4) instrumentation shift, i.e. a change in approach, may quite unspecifically result in improvements; (5) regression to the mean alone can be responsible for the observed change.

The anecdotal case study, therefore, cannot be used to explain the aetiology of a disease, or to assess the effectiveness of the therapy given.

The Intensive Design Approach

An intensive design as opposed to an extensive one (with many subjects), mainly studies replications, or events, in a single subject instead of the same response in several subjects. The intensive design has also been called the $N=1$ experimental design or the small-sample design. Instead of giving different treatments to different groups of subjects, as in the extensive design, the same

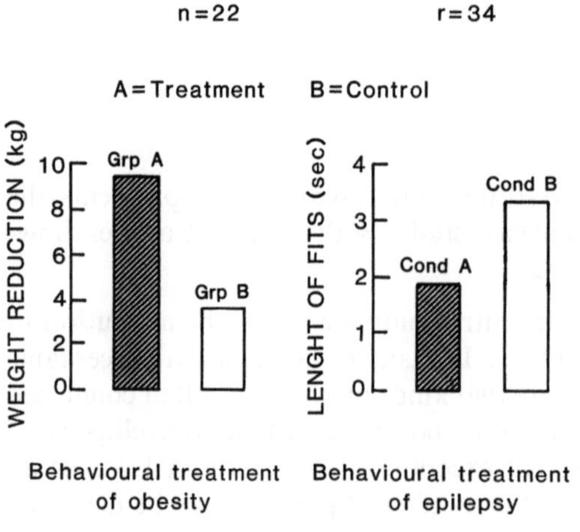

Fig. 1. Examples of results from extensive and intensive designs

subject is studied in different conditions, either in different periods of time or on parallel occasions within a period of time.

The results from a group study (on obesity; Öst and Götestam 1976) and those from an intensive study (on epilepsy; Melin et al. 1983) are depicted in Fig. 1 for comparison. In the group study the number of subjects was 22, randomly assigned to a treatment ($n=11$) or a control group ($n=11$). In the intensive study, the number of observations or replications was 34, divided into treatment sessions ($n=17$) and control sessions ($n=17$; in fact there were 34 control sessions and 17 treatment sessions, not all shown here).

In the group study differences could be tested by independent t test, and in the intensive study, dependent t tests could be used. Analysis of variance, which is often used in group studies, can also be used in an intensive design (Gentile et al. 1972).

The oldest type of intensive design uses a crossover, such as in trials of several drugs where all patients receive all treatments. Examination of some examples of intensive designs shows that there are two main types: (1) replication designs, which often have reversibility as a possible or desired component, although some do not need it; and (2) multiple-baseline designs, which are more useful for the study of non-reversible events such as are often the goal of psychotherapy (psychotherapy should lead to permanent changes).

Replication Designs

The B Design. This is the same as the anecdotal case study, except that it is described using intensive design vocabulary. The only improvement is that the therapy process is assessed empirically (see Fig. 2).

The AB Design. The addition to this design is a baseline period which enables study of the effect of the start of contact with the therapist. As the problem is often assessed by the therapist, this often gives him or her some control over the problem; sometimes this design is inadvertantly called "assessment therapy" as it has therapeutic gains. Two examples (both including a follow-up although this is not necessary in the AB design) show the course of process of therapy. The first is a study of an obsessive case (Lindquist and Götestam 1975). During baseline assessment, the patient reported that the assessment immediately reduced the time with obsessions to about a tenth. With a thought-stopping procedure the obsessions were totally removed (Fig. 3). In a case of severe anxiety (Götestam et al. 1974), an operant procedure reduced anxiety and increased the patient's ability to be alone (Fig. 4).

ABA Design. When some behaviour or problem is under environmental control and it is not a question of learning or knowing a new behaviour, replication can improve the design and can show that the behaviour in question is in fact under such environmental control. In an experiment with an epileptic boy (Melin et al. 1983), it was clear that it was possible to control his epileptic EEG activity externally using an auditory stimulus (Fig. 5).

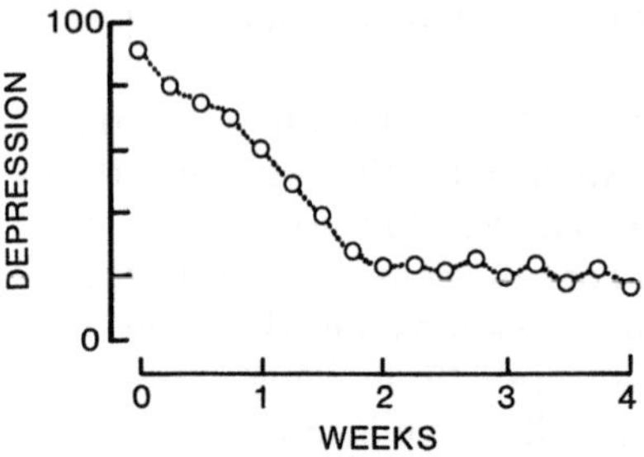

Fig. 2. Example of results from a replication (B) design: study of a depressed patient

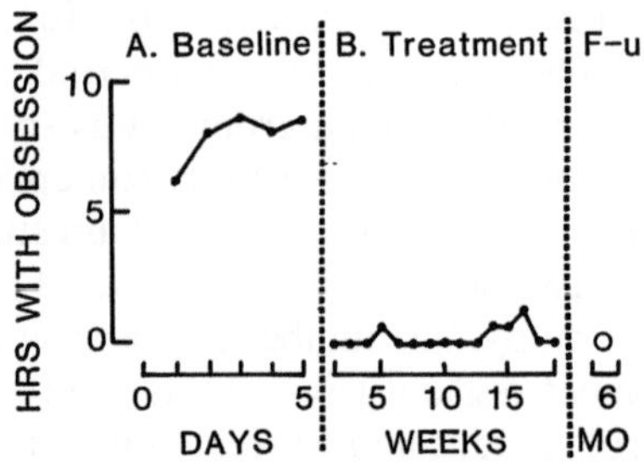

Fig. 3. Example of results from a replication (AB) design; study of an obsessive patient

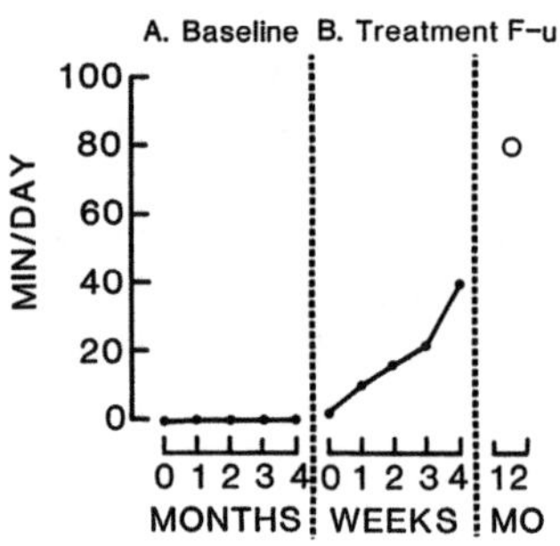

Fig. 4. Example of results from a replication (AB) design; study of a case of severe anxiety

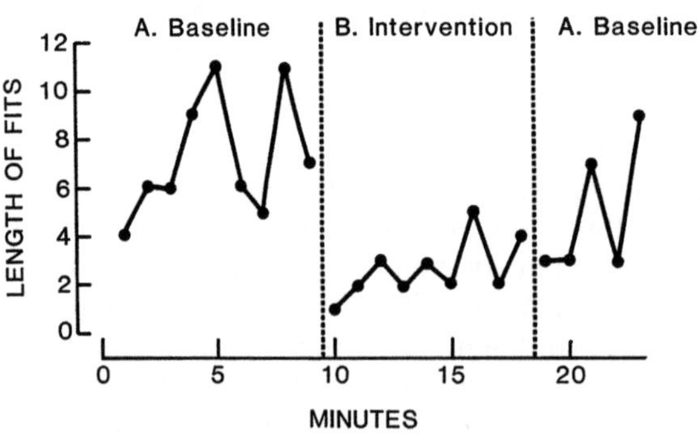

Fig. 5. Example of results from a replication (ABA) design; study of an epileptic boy

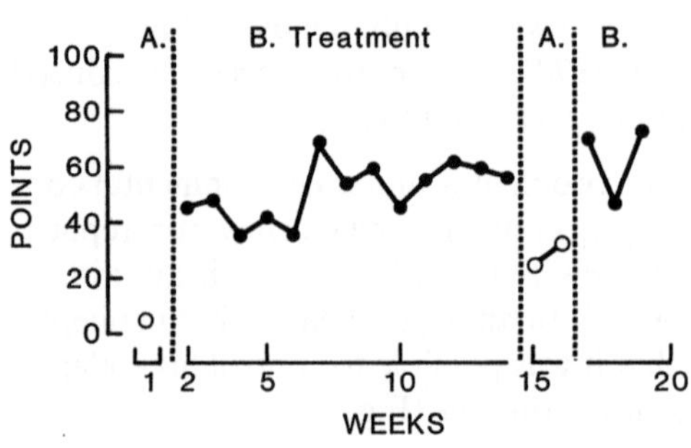

Fig. 6. Example of results from a replication (ABAB) design; study of a schizophrenic man

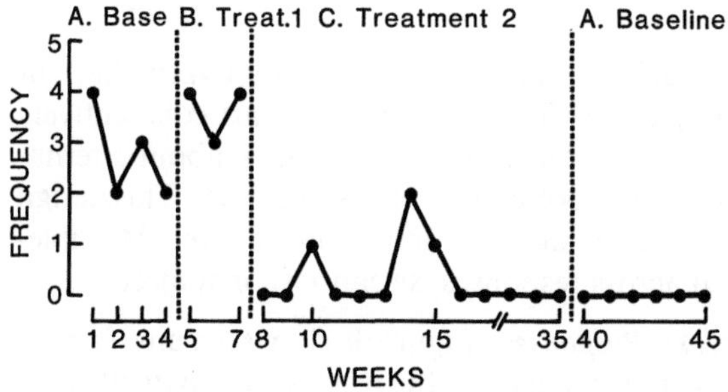

Fig. 7. Example of results from a replication (ABC) design; aggressive behaviour in a schizophrenic woman

ABAB Design. In a case such as that above, it is more appropriate to conclude the experiment with a new treatment phase in order to leave the patient with as much experience and reinforcement of the problem reduction as possible. Thus, an ABAB design might be preferred to an ABA design in most instances. A token economy improved the activity of a schizophrenic man, but only during the active treatment phases (Fig. 6).

ABC Design. When one intervention is not effective enough, another can be tried consecutively. This constitutes an ABC design. In Fig. 7 the frequency of aggressive spells in a schizophrenic woman are shown in relation to different treatment strategies. After about 1 year, the imposed contingencies could be taken away without relapse in aggressive behaviour (Öst et al. 1976). Figure 8 shows increased eye contact and reduced lip biting occurred when social skills were trained with video-assisted feedback (Öst et al. 1976). Reversals are also possible in ABC designs, for instance ABAC or ABCAD sequences.

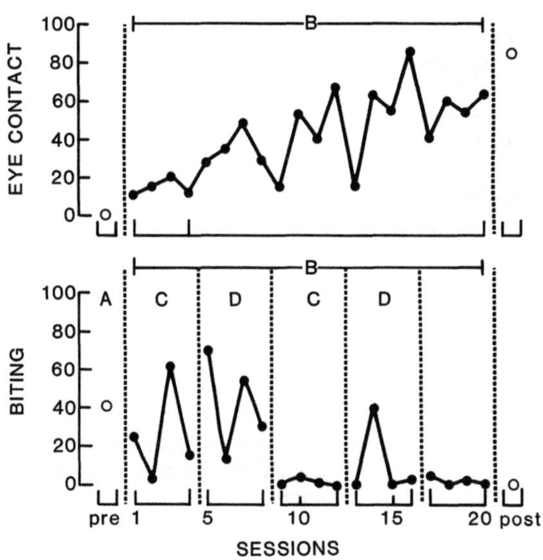

Fig. 8. Example of results from a replication (ABC) design; social skills training in a schizophrenic

Multiple-Baseline Designs

A multiple-baseline design has different baselines for different variables, but all the variables are studied in parallel. The interventions start consecutively rather than simultaneously to enable conclusions to be drawn about alternative explanations (such as other things occurring at the same time). This design is not dependent on behaviour reverting to a pretreatment level. Multiple-baseline designs can be applied across responses, situations, or subjects.

Multiple-Baseline Design Across Responses. Figure 9 shows results from a study of the effects of environmental changes on the responses of patients with senile dementia (Melin and Götestam 1981). Changes in the physical environment, mealtime routines and the availability of activity material substantially improved communication, eating behaviour and activity, respectively.

Multiple-Baseline Design Across Situations. Figure 10 shows results from a study of the reality orientation of patients with senile dementia across situations (Götestam 1987), where situational control was achieved for time and room orientation but not for orientation to person.

Multiple-Baseline Design Across Subjects. In Figure 11, it can be seen that temperature feedback showed the clearest effect in treatment of erythrophobia (Götestam et al. 1976) across subjects.

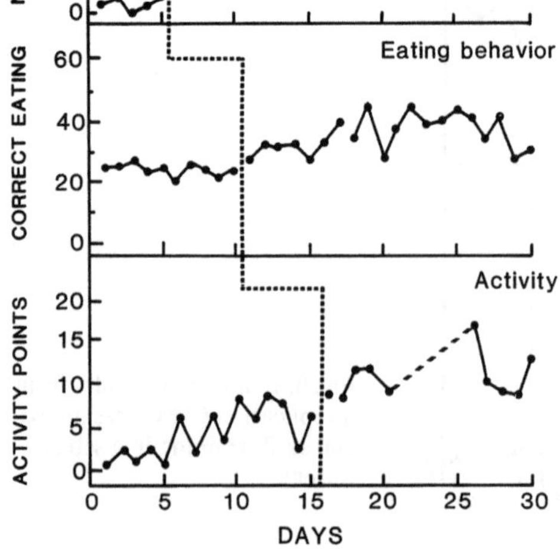

Fig. 9. Example of results from a study using a multiple-baseline design across responses

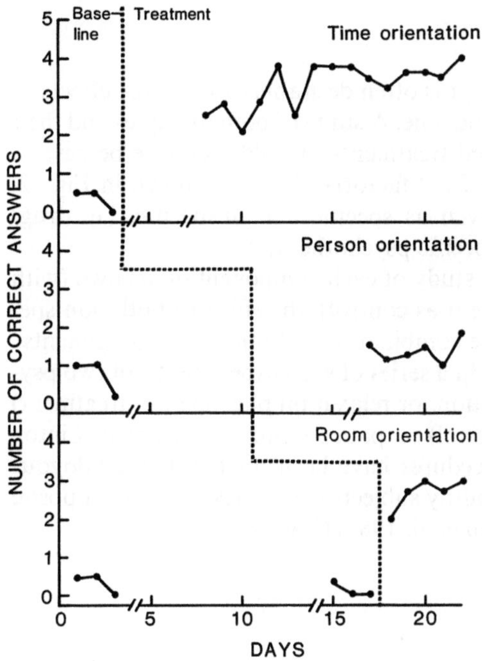

Fig. 10. Example of results from a study using a multiple-baseline design across situations

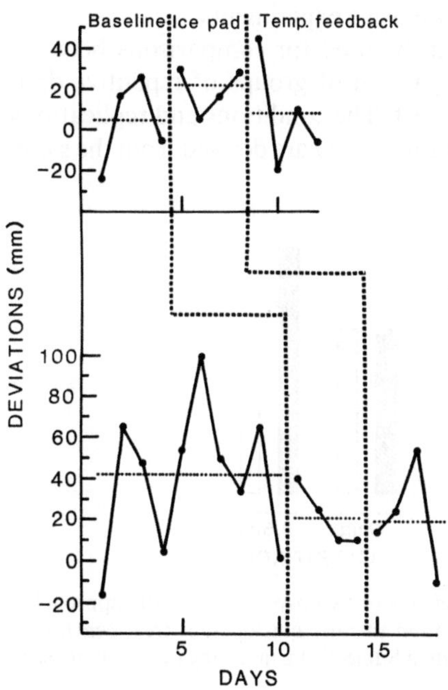

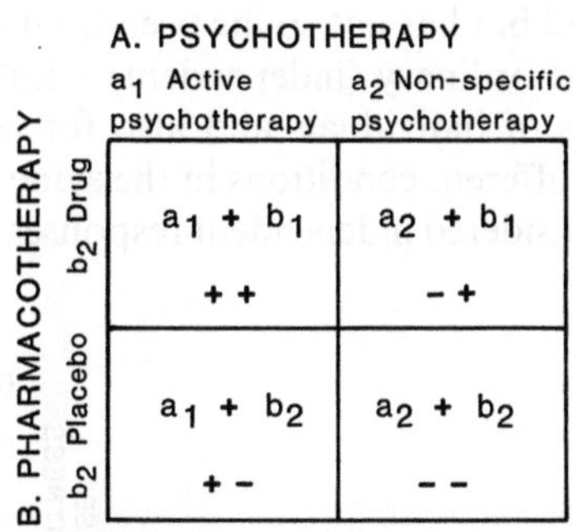

Fig. 12. General outline of a study with a 2×2 factorial design; mixed treatment with pharmacotherapy and psychotherapy

Fig. 11. Example of results from a study using a multiple-baseline design across subjects

Mixed Treatments

In the study of different treatments it is often desirable to study the effects of drugs and psychotherapy at the same time. A study of both therapies and their combination (i.e. a design for mixed treatments), would therefore be best. A general outline for a study with a 2×2 factorial design is shown in Fig. 12. Both treatment modalities are given as specific and unspecific, i.e. drug/placebo and psychotherapy/non-specific psychotherapy.

This kind of design enables the study of each component on its own (with the placebo or non-specific treatment as control), the effect of both non-specific (placebo) components, and the combination of both active components.

Figure 13 compares the effects, in a series of such experiments, of two psychotherapeutic approaches (relaxation, or relaxation plus operant treatment) and medication (placebo of flupentixol) on patients with chronic pain (Linton and Götestam 1984). Similar procedures have been used in two analogous studies of experimental pain on healthy subjects with, unexpectedly, opposite results (Anseth et al. 1985; Berntzen et al. 1985) (Fig. 14).

Statistical Methods

The analysis of variance is a robust statistical method which can be applied both to intensive designs (Gentile et al. 1973) and to the factorial designs mentioned in the section on mixed treatments. Covariance analysis is also a feasible method but has not so far been tried in intensive experiments.

The ordinary (independent) *t* test can be used for comparisons between groups of individuals and also for comparison of groups of repetitive data from different conditions in the same subject. The conditions and replications are considered independent responses although they are derived from the same

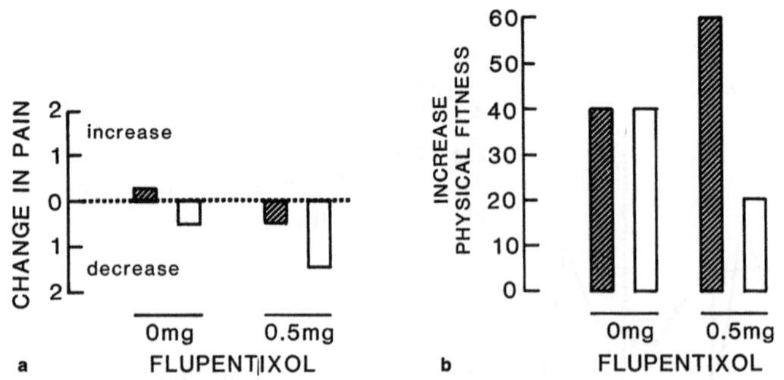

Fig. 13 a, b. Results of a study comparing the effects of two psychotherapeutic approaches (□, *AR*, relaxation therapy; □, *AR+OP*, relaxation therapy plus operant treatment), with placebo or flupentixol, in patients in chronic pain. **a** Subjective pain rating (VAS); **b** physical exercise test

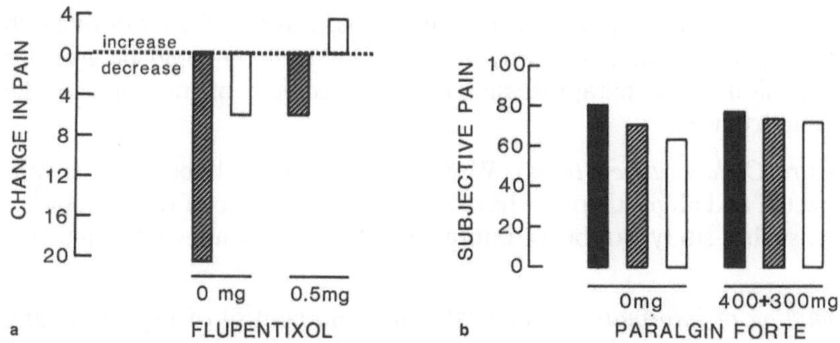

Fig. 14 a, b. Results of two studies of pain perception. **a** Anseth et al. (1985), on the influence of flupentixol; 2 × 2 design. □, with relaxation; □, control. **b** Berntzen et al. (1985), on the influence of instructional intervention; 2 × 3 design; ■, no intervention; ▨, with positive intervention; □ with negative intervention

individual. Dependent *t* tests may be used in comparisons of paired observations. Time-series analysis is also a useful statistical tool, especially when the therapy process is studied and several replicated assessments are made (Tryon 1982).

Future Priorities

To improve psychotherapy research in the future, some procedures can be advocated.

Better Control Conditions. As it is never possible to prove the null hypothesis, the use of comparison groups other than placebo (or unspecific treatment) should be considered. When a new treatment is compared to a well-known and empirically effective treatment, it is rather difficult to establish a significant difference. Thus, the new treatment might be considered to be "effective" on these grounds. It is therefore of importance to have a placebo group as a more safe comparison. Significant differences are then necessary to give the new treatment approval. Such a strategy will probably reduce the number of new drugs of inferior quality that are introduced, and similarly psychotherapies. Random assignment to conditions is also of utmost importance, as otherwise no proof of effectiveness can be obtained.

Assessment of Independent Variables. When a study is performed and a therapy is applied, we know that some patients do not do as they are asked. From drug trials, we know that patient compliance is far from perfect and there is reason to believe that this is an even more pronounced problem in psychotherapy research. Assessments to ascertain that the therapy procedure has really been applied are therefore an important aid in the improvement of therapy research.

Training. Training in clinical treatment methods, and specifically in research methodology and design, is greatly needed. This training could be given to both professionals and paraprofessionals. The specificity of training is of the utmost importance.

Multicentre Collaborative Studies. When a multicentre collaboration is skilfully directed and all participants have sufficient knowledge of research methodology, such a study can be an improvement on one conducted in a single centre.

Dissemination of Information. The evaluation and control of psychotherapy should be a governmental task. Furthermore, the present knowledge from research reports should be spread much more widely, and this should also be through government agencies. Maybe research on information dissemination would also be worthwile.

References

Anseth E, Berntzen D, Götestam KG (1985) Flupentixol and relaxation in the treatment of laboratory pain: an experimental study. Acta Neurol Scand 71:20–24

Berntzen D, Fors E, Götestam KG (1985) Effect of an analgesic drug (Paralgin forte) upon laboratory pain under different cognitive manipulations. An experimental study. Acta Neurol Scand 72:30–35

Elkin I, Parloff MB, Hadley SW, Autry JH (1985) NIMH treatment of depression collaborative research program: background and research plan. Arch Gen Psychiatry 42:305–316

Gentile JR, Roden AH, Klein RD (1972) An analysis-of-variance model for the intrasubject replication design. J Appl Behav Anal 5:193–198

Götestam KG (1987) Learning versus environmental support for increasing reality orientation in senile demented patients. Eur J Psychiatry (in press)

Götestam KG, Hultman C, Olingdal G (1974) Positiv förstärkning i behandling av kroniskt neurostillstånd (Positive reinforcement in the treatment of a chronic neurosis). Scand J Behav Ther 3:37–44

Götestam KG, Melin L, Olsson B (1976) Behandling av erythrofobi med avkylning och temperaturfeedback (Treatment of erythrophobia with cooling and temperature feedback). Scand J Behav Ther 5:153–159

Kazdin AE (1980) Research design in clinical psychology. Harper and Row, New York

Lindquist M, Götestam KG (1975) Behandling av tvangstankar med tankestopp (Treatment of an obsessive patient with thought stopping). Scand J Behav Ther 4:35–39

Linton SJ, Götestam KG (1984) Integration of pharmacological and psychological treatment of chronic pain patients: a preliminary study. Nord Psykiatr Tidsskr 38:31–34

Melin L, Götestam KG (1981) The effects of rearranging ward routines on communication and eating behaviors of psychogeriatric patients. J Appl Behav Anal 14:24–28

Melin L, Götestam KG, Sjödén P-O (1983) Effect of auditive stimulation on epileptic EEG activity. Epilepsia 24:219–224

Öst L-G, Götestam KG (1976) Behavioral and pharmacological treatment for obesity: an experimental comparison. Addict Behav 1:331–338

Öst L-G, Melin L, Götestam KG (1976) A token economy for chronic schizophrenic patients. Scand J Psychol 17:272–282

Tryon WW (1982) A simplified time-series analysis for evaluating treatment interventions. J Appl Behav Anal 15:423–429

The Evaluation of Sex Therapy: Some Methodological Considerations

J. Bancroft[1]

The number of controlled studies of sex therapy is still relatively small (for reviews see Jehu 1979; Marks 1981b; Bancroft 1983), but the prevailing impression from them is a lack of any convincingly demonstrated superiority of one method over another. Trends, when they occur, tend to be weak and not always in the same direction.

The main conclusions that have been drawn from these studies have depended on the absence of demonstrable differences in outcome between different practical approaches to treatment, e.g. two therapists are no better than one, or daily treatment sessions are no more effective than weekly. It is important to remember that whereas replication of a positive finding is significant, repeating a negative result means very little.

One study stands out as having clearly significant treatment effects (Carney et al. 1978). In this study, which involved women with sexual unresponsiveness and their partners, drug treatment was combined with sex therapy. All couples received sex therapy (half on a weekly basis and half monthly) and half of the women received testosterone (10 mg sublingually daily) and the other half diazepam (10 mg daily). Although there were no differences in outcome between the weekly and monthly regimes, the women receiving testosterone did significantly better on a number of key outcome variables. Unfortunately, two subsequent studies (Mathews et al. 1983; Dow 1983) using a similar design with the important exception that placebo rather than diazepam was involved, failed to find any superiority of testosterone over placebo. In fact, Mathews et al. (1983) found some effects to be superior with placebo. Should we be looking for explanations based on placebo-induced mechanisms or are these results instead an example of experimental error?

My uncertainties about this crucial question increased when we started to analyse a later study (Bancroft et al. 1986) of men with erectile problems and loss of sexual interest. We used a very similar design to that of Carney et al. (1978). Men with sexual dysfunction received sex therapy together with their partners. Half of them also received testosterone undecanoate 160 mg daily, the other half placebo. We found no main effects of the testosterone, but for a number of variables there was superiority for placebo. It then became appar-

[1] MRC Reproductive Biology Unit, 37 Chalmers Street, Edinburgh EH 3 9EW, United Kingdom

Psychological Treatment of Mental Illness
Edited by R. J. Daly and E. A. Sand

ent that in spite of randomization the two treatment groups (i.e. hormone and placebo) were different before treatment on a number of variables with prognostic significance. Some of these pretreatment differences reached statistical significance.

The results of this study are therefore uninterpretable but they raised the question of what might have happened if the bias had operated in the other direction and we had found significant superiority of the active treatment. Would we have published these results as positive? To what extent has this happened in other reported treatment studies?

In looking at the literature on treatment outcome research in sex therapy, we found three principal ways of dealing with any pretreatment group difference.

1. Ignore them – several studies have not commented on the comparison of pretreatment characteristics.

2. Report a lack of statistical difference between groups prior to treatment. This usually involves an arbitrary collection of patient variables, and the implication is that the absence of any significant difference means that there is no problem. The fact that a bias falls on the right side of the 5% significance levels does not stop it exerting an effect on the results. In how many studies has such a bias operated? In most cases it is not possible to say.

3. Use analysis of covariance to deal with pretreatment imbalance. Analysis of covariance has gained a certain respectability in the treatment literature as a way of dealing with this problem. We believe that this is based on false premises. The principal use for covariance analysis in randomized experiments is to increase precision by removing from the variability of the outcome measure that part which is due to its relationship with the covariate. According to Lord (1967) "there is simply no logical or statistical procedure that can make proper allowances for uncontrolled pre-existing differences between groups." Analysis of covariance is a delicate instrument and if certain conditions are not met may lead to spurious results, either positive or negative.

In spite of these negative and weak research findings, most people working in sex therapy have the clinical impression that it is effective, whilst at the same time realising that some patients respond much more readily than others. This source of variance, the prognostic characteristics of a patient or couple, is probably far greater than those sources that tend to be controlled in experimental studies, e.g. one or two therapists, frequency of treatment sessions.

At the present time, it would be very difficult to control for the key prognostic factors because our understanding of such factors is negligible, due mainly to a paucity of research aimed at identifying them. It seems that treatment outcome research has been much more popular with both researchers and funding agencies, than the less exciting studies of prognosis without which the treatment studies may not be fruitful.

This comment is of course not restricted to sex therapy. It applies to the bulk of research into behavioural psychotherapy. It is a serious question whether much of treatment outcome research in behaviour therapy has up to now been a waste of time. There are two important qualifications to this question: (1) the use of the patient as his own control, which avoids most of these problems; unfortunately, the use of a crossover design is only applicable to treatments which have a reversible effect, which excludes most types of psychotherapy, behavioural or otherwise. (2) the tradition of behaviour therapy has been based on a modification of relatively specific behaviours directly influenced by the tretment method. The control of obsessional behaviour is such an example. It is noteworthy that the literature on modification of obsessional behaviour is relatively consistent, with positive results (for review see Marks 1981a). The treatment of sexual problems, by contrast, is dealing with highly complex interpersonal processes, and the improvement of sexual function usually depends upon changes in this interpersonal component. The treatment of agoraphobia comes midway between these two relative extremes. In this respect sex therapy is closer to non-behavioural evocative psychotherapy than most forms of behavioural treatment.

Another way of looking at this dimension is to consider how close the behavioural change being measured is to the focal effects of the treatment method. With obsessional behaviour, treatment is usually focused directly on the symptoms and changes in the symptoms are measured. With sex therapy, outcome is usually judged by assessing changes in sexual response when the treatment method is focused more on communication and other inter- or intrapersonal processes.

There are therefore two basic requirements that need to be met before controlled outcome evaluation of sex therapy is likely to be productive. First, we need appropriate measures of variables which have been shown to have prognostic significance. Some of these are likely to be directly related to the specific treatment method. For example, most sex therapy focuses to a considerable extent on communication between the couple. There should therefore be appropriate measures of communication. The second requirement is that in treatment studies, groups should be balanced for the key prognostic variables. One cannot rely on randomization to achieve this unless large numbers are involved or one's conclusions are based on a series of replicating studies. With treatment research of this kind, it is inevitable that relatively small numbers are involved. Even so, outcome research is extremely time consuming and there is an understandable desire to draw as many conclusions as possible from a single study. Thus, if we are comparing two treatment methods, one focusing mainly on communication, the other on anxiety reduction, we should not only have measures of both communication and anxiety, but we should ensure that our treatment groups are balanced for both variables.

Obviously there are severe limits to the number of variables that can be balanced in this way. It is therefore of the utmost importance that we obtain good research evidence of the relative prognostic significance of different variables so that we can choose accordingly and maximize the balancing of the sources of variance in our design.

I am not prepared to embark on further treatment outcome studies in sex therapy until we have more evidence on this point. Hawton and Catalan (1986) have made a useful start identifying prognostic variables such as the quality of the general relationship. But particular attention to analysing the process of sex therapy is required so that the most important focal effects can be identified and relevant patient characteristics measured. Communication and anxiety reduction have already been mentioned but there are likely to be others of comparable importance.

References

Bancroft J (1983) Human sexuality and its problems. Churchill Livingstone, Edinburgh, pp 257–263

Bancroft J, Dickerson M, Fairburn CJ, Gray J, Greenwood J, Stevenson N, Warner P (1986). Sex therapy outcome research: a reappraisal of methodology. Psychol Med 16:851–863

Carney A, Bancroft J, Mathews A (1978) Combination of hormonal and psychological treatment for female sexual unresponsiveness: a comparative study. Br J Psychiatry 133:339–346

Dow MGT (1983) A controlled comparative evaluation of conjoint counselling and self-help behavioural treatment for sexual dysfunction. Unpublished PhD Thesis, University of Glasgow

Hawton K, Catalan J (1986) Prognostic factors in sex therapy. Behav Res Ther 24:377–385

Jehu D (1979) Sexual dysfunction: a behavioural approach to causation, assessment and treatment. Wiley, Chichester

Marks I (1981a) Review of behavioural psychotherapy I: obsessive-compulsive disorders. Am J Psychiatry 138:584–592

Marks I (1981b) Review of behavioural psychotherapy II: sexual disorders. Am J Psychiatry 138:750–756

Mathews A, Whitehead A, Kellet J (1983) Psychological and hormonal factors in the treatment of female sexual dysfunction. Psychol Med 13:83–92

Subject Index

MIX
Papier aus verantwortungsvollen Quellen
Paper from responsible sources
FSC® C105338

If you have any concerns about our products,
you can contact us on
ProductSafety@springernature.com

In case Publisher is established outside the EU,
the EU authorized representative is:
Springer Nature Customer Service Center GmbH
Europaplatz 3, 69115 Heidelberg, Germany

Printed by Libri Plureos GmbH
in Hamburg, Germany